Yin Yoga for EVERY Body

Sue Blei

ISBN: 9781728652375
ISBN-13:

This book is dedicated to all the students who inspire me. I humbly thank you for allowing me to guide you.

Table of Contents

Chapter Six

Chapter Seven

Chapter Eight

INTRODUCTION

The Steps of My Personal Yoga Path

For me, Yin Yoga is the most personal and intimate style of yoga that I practice. Yin allows me to focus my thoughts and attentions inward. There is time to listen to my thoughts and my body during a Yin practice. Because I feel Yin is so personal, I would like to share a little of my yoga journey with you.

Yoga has always been an evolving and ever-changing exploration for me. Sometimes it is a purely physical journey. Sometimes it is a spiritual journey. I suppose that most often, it is a combination of the two. It seems that the more I practice, the more I change and grow.

I'm not usually good with dates, but I do remember when I started practicing yoga. I remember because, just a few months later, our country was hit with a horrific terrorist attack. I had just dropped my son off at preschool and I remember there was talk on the radio about airplanes and buildings on fire. I felt a little confused, as if I could not comprehend what I was hearing. I remember not wanting to process such bad news and I turned the station.

When I got home, I felt stressed from what was on the radio. I still had no idea of the scope of what was unfolding. I got my mat out and began to practice yoga. In that moment on that morning, my practice gave me a sense of peace. Eventually, I began to let go of hearing about what I thought was a terrible plane accident. I dropped into a space of being present and calm. My mat was a place that was safe.

That sense of peace and serenity was shattered when I received a phone call telling me to turn on the news.

I, along with the rest of the world, was watching the unthinkable. What I couldn't process in the car with the radio was in living color on my TV as I watched the news. There was still so much confusion in my mind. Who would do this? Why would someone do this?

The events of September 11th changed all of our lives. I knew a different world before that day. We lost a level of trust in the world we didn't even know we were taking for granted. Our sense of safety changed in a profound and permanent way.

My yoga journey took a turn on that day. I understood that my practice was a place that made sense of a senseless world. My yoga practice became a source of quiet solace. While I felt hyperaware of my surroundings off the mat, I could center on peace in the moment on my mat.

I remember planting flowers outside just a day or two after 9/11. A plane flew overhead. I was alarmed because all flights were grounded immediately after the attack. I felt a twinge of panic that was a new sensation for me. I had to remind myself that I live near a military base and it was probably just a military plane. I had to repeat to myself that I am safe. I am thankful that yoga was already a part of my journey on that day. The peace we cultivate on the mat is always within.

My journey took another turn when I decided to go through yoga teacher training. I have always been happiest when helping others. Early in my career I was a counselor and later became an elementary school teacher. These were great avenues to help people grow but I felt that yoga would be even more fulfilling.

Yoga teacher training widened the path of my journey. While I had a strong yoga practice before training, I did not explore yoga outside of what I heard in class. The classes I attended mainly focused on alignment and very rarely would a teacher speak to yoga philosophy. I knew there was more to learn about yoga than what I already knew and yoga teacher training opened that door.

While I learned how to perfect alignment in yoga poses during training, I also learned about ways to explore yoga philosophy. I learned about some of the ancient texts on which the physical practice of yoga was founded. I love the story in ***The Bhagavad Gita***. It taught me so much about duty and dharma. I have read the **Gita** several times now and I feel like I keep finding little nuggets of wisdom with each new read. This learning phase continues to be an active and enjoyable journey outside of teacher training.

Most people who go through yoga teacher training say they experience a personal change. We are exposed to concepts like the Yamas and Niyamas in ***The Yoga Sutras of Patanjali***. These concepts are all about living life as a good yogi. The Yamas are moral and ethical guidelines sometimes referred to as the five restraints. The Niyamas are internal practices known as the five observances or duties. I think about how I apply the Yamas and Niyamas to my practice, to teaching, and to people around me. I am reminded to live with kindness and compassion. The yoga teacher training part of my journey has encouraged me behave like a better person.

When I completed yoga teacher training, I immediately started to teach yoga a few times a week. I kept my job as a school teacher for the first few years I taught yoga. If you are a school teacher or are close to a teacher, you know that this can be a very stressful position. You would think that teaching at school for eight to ten hours would make it impossible to go teach a yoga class or add anything to an already full plate.

What I found on my yoga journey is that teaching

yoga uplifted me. I may have had a headache from a stressful day of meetings, testing, and data disaggregation as a school teacher only to teach a yoga class and actually feel better after teaching. It is such a wonderful thing to be able to share yoga with others!

Most of my yoga journey as a teacher and student has centered around Yang style yoga. Yang was all I knew in the beginning. During those years my practice and teaching was limited to Yang styles like traditional Hatha yoga or Vinyasa yoga. My very favorite style to teach and practice came to be Vinyasa which is a fast paced yoga style that moves with the breath.

Yang yoga focuses on strengthening and stretching muscles. Yang yoga is precise in the way we arrange the body into poses. There is an order to Yang a class that allows the body to warm up and strengthen leading up to a peak pose or series. There is a cool down element at the end of a Yang practice that tends to stretch the muscles which have strengthened during the class. There may be so much instruction during a Yang class that there is little silence from the instructor.

A new teacher to my studio suggested adding a Yin class. As she described the class to me, it sounded really dull. I did not think anyone would want to take a class where you hang out in a pose for three or more minutes. In this fast paced world, who can get their mind to quiet for that long?

I almost passed on adding the class to our schedule. The teacher was so passionate that I reluctantly added the class to our schedule. I thought I would add it to our list of classes and then take it off the schedule after a few weeks when no one showed up. I did not even give the class a full hour time slot. I had very low expectations for Yin Yoga.

I took the first class and was immediately blown away. I almost missed this part of my yoga journey without even giving it a chance. The class whizzed by so fast that I was not ready for it to end. Thank goodness for that lovely yoga instructor. If I had not been convinced by her excitement for Yin, I would not be writing this book today.

In that first Yin class I saw a different side of yoga. My mind was able to settle in a different way than I find in a Yang style class. When I am strengthening my muscles and finding proper yoga alignment, I feel like my mind is present centered because I am so aware of my body and my breath. I am thinking about how I can find that balance between strength and comfort while building the best alignment possible in my body. Focusing so intently on my Yang practice leaves little space for my mind to wander off. Yang yoga offers my mind a different way of being in the now than during Yin yoga.

There is a certain ease in Yin. The muscles soften but there is still sensation in the body. The softening of the muscles along with the amount of time spent in Yin poses allowed my mind to calm in a fresh new way. I felt like poses and meditation were beginning to come together in a new and unexpected approach. During Yin I feel as if I have several small windows of time to drop into short meditations. It seems as the Yin practice goes on, the easier it is to drop in with both a willing body and a meditative mind.

My body experienced poses in a whole new light during Yin. Pigeon Pose has always been a favorite Yang pose of mine. In Pigeon I will arrange my body so that I feel the most sensation as I find my edge in the pose at the beginning of the posture. This pose becomes Swan in a Yin practice. I arrange my body in a different way for Swan because holding the pose and letting go of muscular strength makes this pose feel different. Swan pose develops very intense sensations for my hips the longer I hold in stillness. I have to remember to release into the posture and embrace the sensations during a long Yin hold. My body feels different even though it is in the same general shape in the two different yoga styles. How wonderful to discover new things about my body and my practice.

I would like to share what I have learned and witnessed so far on my Yin Yoga journey. My journey is not complete and I'm happy to say that I learn new things about Yin all the time. I gain more insight into how others may experience Yin physically and mentally as more and more people tell me how they have been affected by a Yin practice.

PHILOSOPHY OF YIN YOGA

Just about every Yin book touches on Yin Yoga philosophy. Some Yin books will give you more information on certain aspects like meridian theory or chakras. My main focus in this book is to help you find a space for your mind and body during Yin poses. I will just scratch the surface of some of the Yin philosophy in the next few paragraphs. If your interest is in philosophy is piqued, please explore these topics further in your personal yoga journey.

Yin and Yang exists in everything. Yin and Yang characteristics are opposites. You must have one to see the distinction of the other. The Yin/Yang symbol is a circle of black and white with a dot of the opposite color in each segment. The black color represents Yin while the white color represents Yang. The dot of the opposing color reminds us that there is a little Yin within Yang and a little Yang present in Yin. One cannot exist without the other.

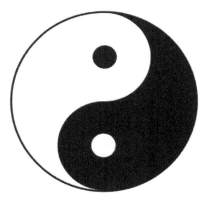

Yin is associated with being dark and cool like the North side of the mountain. Yang is warm and bright like the South side of the mountain. You might expect that Yin is connected to the quiet winter season while Yang connects to the busy season of summer. A person with Yin dominated qualities might be described as sensitive, nurturing, intuitive, quiet, relaxed, or introverted. Yang minded people might be described as excited, rational, enthusiastic, outgoing, or logical.

Too much Yin or too much Yang can cause an imbalance. A person who may possess excessive Yin might feel depressed, gain weight easily, or linger over past events. One with too much Yang might feel anxious, hyperactive, reactive, or emotionless. Yoga is one tool that can help bring a person back into balance.

Some Yin practices are guided by balancing meridian lines in the body. Meridians were first described in Traditional Chinese Medicine (TCM). Meridian lines are rivers or channels of energy that are present in the body. These lines travel through precise parts of the body. If you have ever seen a meridian map for an acupuncture therapist, you know there are many points on the body that influence energy flow.

Your energy in TCM is known as Chi. You may sometimes see chi spelled qi. When chi is out of balance, the body or mind is out of balance. Energy is constantly moving around the body. We do not always notice right away when the imbalance begins. During Yin you have the opportunity to explore your thoughts and your physical body to detect imbalance.

Each meridian is associated with an organ. The Yin meridians are associated with solid organs and Yang meridians with hollow organs. Each Yin meridian is paired with a Yang meridian. Yin Yoga focuses on twelve meridians or six pairs of meridians.

I'm writing this book in the fall so I'll share an example of the organ pairs associated with this season. The lungs and large intestine are the meridian lines connected to autumn. The lung is the Yin organ while the large intestine is the Yang organ. This pair is symbolic of breathing in new possibilities or chi (lungs) and letting go of waste or things that no longer serve you (large intestine).

The meridians have a specific location on the body. The lung meridian begins inside the body at the stomach. It travels down to the large intestine then back up past the stomach, across the diaphragm, and then breaks into the lungs. The meridian comes back together and travels up to the throat then breaks again toward the shoulders ending at the end of the thumbs.

The large intestine meridian begins at the end of the index finger. It travels along the finger, up the arm to the shoulder, then to the side of the neck, up the face and over the top lip.

A fun activity is tracing the meridian lines on your body. You can see several different videos on YouTube that explain how to trace your meridian lines. You may feel a shift in energy after completing the tracing.

If you teach a Yin class or take a Yin class where the lung/large intestine organ pair is the focus, the poses will put stress on these meridian lines. When these meridians are balanced you may feel your thinking is clearer, self-esteem increases, organization is improved, and overall happiness increases. After each pose of the class, you will pause for a moment to allow the chi to move around your body. There is an example of a class centered around the lung/large intestine meridian pair in the Yin Yoga Sequence section at the end of this book.

Yin classes may be inspired by aligning chakras. The main seven chakras are described as wheels or discs of energy. These seven chakras begin at the base of the spine and travel up the spine all the way to the crown of the head. Each chakra represents specific colors, elements, and feelings. The first chakra is red and follows the colors of the rainbow up the spine ending with the purple chakra at the top of the head.

Just like the meridian lines the chakras want to be in balance. Energy is in balance when there is not too much or too little of the chakra chi in the body. Imbalance in the chakras can manifest as negative physical and emotional changes.

Let's look at the first chakra as an example. The Muladhara Chakra is also called the Root Chakra. It is located at the base of the spine. The color of the Root Chakra is red. The element related to the Root Chakra is earth. When the Root Chakra is in balance a person feels rooted and grounded which may be translated into feeling safe and secure. When the Root Chakra is blocked a person may react from a place of fear and insecurity.

There is a sequence inspired by the chakras in this book. The sequence touches on all seven chakras and gives a brief explanation of each chakra.

Meridians and chakras can be a great source of inspiration when you are putting a class together for yourself or students.

YIN YOGA VS YANG YOGA

The way Yin yoga is taught and the way Yin yoga is experienced is very different than Yang yoga. As a teacher and practitioner of Yang yoga for many years, the difference for me was tremendous. I think it took me at least a year of teaching Yin before I really surrendered and became comfortable with the differences in teaching a Yin style class.

In Yin yoga there is no exact place for your body in a pose. The idea is to find the general shape of the pose. There is a very broad range of how a body looks. Think more about what part of the body is targeted. Focus on feeling sensation rather than arranging your body for an Instagram photo. Different bodies can appear to be in slightly different shapes or even wildly different shapes and still target the same area.

You will find many ways to arrange the body into the general shape of the pose in the descriptions of the postures later in this book. The posture descriptions guide a person by using props or adjusting the parts of the body to feel sensation that is appropriate for their body. It is important to be respectful and compassionate to each person's experience in the pose. There is no wrong way to do a pose as long as the body is in a safe position and feels sensation in the targeted area.

As the body moves in to the general shape, you are bringing awareness to physical feelings. It is up to the practitioner to decide what feels just right. Only the yogi can decide what shape is correct by listening inward.

We can think about different bodies in Swan Pose. In Swan a person with very open hips may place the shin parallel to the top of the mat while easily draping the body forward. A body that feels tight in the hips may look totally different. Tight hips can be assisted by using props like a blanket or bolster under the hip or thigh. The tight body may also want to have a bolster under their chest rather than bringing the upper body all the way to the floor. While the two bodies are feeling sensation in the hips, they may appear very different on the outside. All versions of the pose are perfect and appropriate for the person performing the pose.

Along the lines of a general shape is the notion that there are no adjustments in Yin yoga. It is a hands off approach for the instructor. The teacher may give verbal cues or even ask questions directly to a particular student to guide the student into the pose. This felt so strange to someone like me who was accustomed to tweaking students' poses with a gentle hand. I still catch myself wanting to move a person just a bit when I teach Yin.

Take Swan Pose again. In a Yang style class, an instructor may give you a fabulous adjustment by placing the hands on the hips and gently pressing down. In a Yin style class, the instructor may use words to guide a practitioner deeper without laying a hand on the body. The instructor may begin by asking, "How do you feel in the pose?" From the answer the student gives, the instructor will follow up with more questions and suggestions until the student comes into a place where they feel a physical change without using muscular strength.

It takes a little more time to allow yogis to come into the perfect expression on their own. The good news is that there is plenty of time to verbally guide a student. Once the instructor has a sound knowledge of props and how to use verbal cues, it is pretty easy to get a student into a space where they are able to feel the effects of the pose.

Yin yoga has a meditative quality. The poses are held for much longer periods of time than in a Yang practice. As a Yin teacher it is a challenge for me to stop talking and allow students to simply be in the pose. There are always more cues I could give to divert attention to sensation and awareness. There is an art to allowing silence to fill the space. The intuition for silence grows with time and teaching.

In that silent space yogis are encouraged to stay with the pose and with the moment. As a Yin student I love those moments of quiet. Time seems to fly by in the peaceful stillness. I often feel others begin to move around me as they are coming out of the pose and I cannot recall the instructor cueing us to exit the pose. I feel so settled in mind and body that I often do not hear the instructor cue the class out of the posture.

The quiet meditative aspect can be a real challenge for some people. Most of the Western world praises multi-tasking and a mind that never stops. We commend athletes who train tirelessly for a sport. Meditation takes training too. It takes discipline and dedication to train the mind. Yin yoga is a safe place to start that journey especially for those who are most reluctant. While mindfulness can be a challenge, I think it is just what the world needs.

There are a few techniques that may help an active

mind. Keeping the mind busy by watching the breath may help keep a person grounded during the quiet spaces of a Yin pose. A simple method of using the breath to stay present is to count the breath. The first inhale and exhale cycle is breath one. The next cycle is breath two. Continue to count the breath all the way to ten. When you reach ten, begin to count the breath back down to one. If you lose your place, start over at one.

Scanning the body during a pose can also help anchor the mind during a pose. You may start at the part of the body that feels the most sensation and then allow the mind to expand throughout the body until all parts of the body have been scanned. If you prefer to start in the same location for each pose, you could start at the toes and mentally work your way up to the top of the head.

As a teacher, I remind students throughout the practice how to come back to the present moment and avoid a mind that is constantly on the go. Each cycle of breath can be used as a reminder to be present for a very busy mind.

Another adjustment from Yang yoga to Yin yoga relates to the way we hold muscular energy. Muscles work hard in Yang style yoga. Muscles grow in strength and flexibility. The strength of the muscles helps to support and bring ease to joints.

In Yin yoga the muscles are given time to release. As the body is still, the muscles relax into a state in which connective tissue can begin to stress. Muscles are encouraged to surrender into stillness so that the fascia and connective tissue can do all the work.

The muscles need to be trained to let go. It is the job of the muscles to stay ready to protect the body. In the beginning of the pose you may spend time exploring the attitude of the muscles. The more you bring awareness to the state of the muscles the more you can actively soften the muscles. Over time it will become easier and faster to allow the muscles to soften from their state of action or being on the verge of action.

It takes time for the muscles to really let go. A mindful scan might reveal spaces in the body that remain tight even after it felt like the body was completely relaxed. Scanning throughout the pose may help a student to recognize patterns of tightening specific places. Yin yoga allows time and introspection to come into a space of stillness so the muscles can release.

Yin and Yang differ in many of the pose names. Yin Yoga uses traditional yoga poses in such a different way that the names are often changed. You might know Paschimottanasana as a seated forward fold in a Yang style class. The Yang version of the pose encourages the muscles to stay active as you flex the ankles and reach toward the toes. The Yin style Caterpillar may look like Paschimottanasana but it is a completely different pose. The joints and muscles are relaxed in Caterpillar. The ankles are soft and you might see the toes fall away from one another in Caterpillar. The intention is to stress connective tissue rather than muscles.

You can see the two styles of yoga differ in many ways. I enjoy finding a balance of the two. Some days my body needs the qualities of Yin class while other days a Yang style class will energize my body. The two styles can even be combined by starting a practice with Yang poses and finishing the class with Yin poses. Find your balance.

PROPS TO HELP YOU FIND YOUR WAY INTO THE POSE

For every Yin class I teach I ask students to start with a basic set of props. These basic props for my students are two yoga blocks, a blanket, and a bolster. Regular students have learned which props they tend to use over and over and might modify the basics to fit their body. Students who feel tight might grab several more blocks and a few extra blankets. A yogi may choose to practice Yin with no props at all.

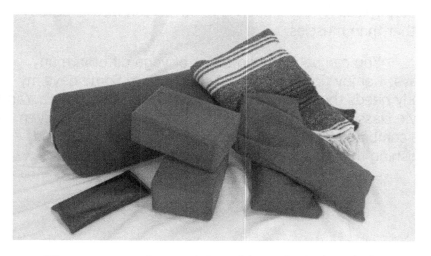

The props we have pictured here include a bolster,

two yoga blocks, a blanket, an eye pillow, and two sandbags.

Some students will adjust the basics to fit their practice. One blanket or one bolster may not be enough to find the general shape of the pose. I've seen students stack several blocks or use three blankets to find the right support. If you are teaching, it's a good idea to have a few extra props nearby just in case a student decides they need it.

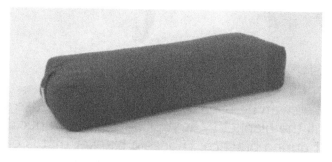

The bolsters I use during practice are 24 inches long, 6 inches high, and 12 inches wide. They weigh a few pounds which can make them tricky to move into certain spaces. The bolsters are pretty firm but soft at the same time. They are ideal if you want soft support. These bolsters have a removable cover. The removable cover is nice because you can pop it into the washer if it gets dirty.

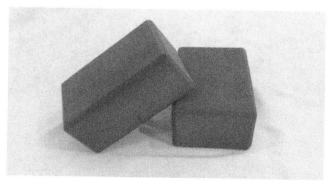

The yoga blocks are made from a very dense foam.

They are solid enough to sit on. Blocks are light and easy to move in place to assist yoga poses. I use the standard size blocks which are 9 inches long, 6 inches wide, and 4 inches thick.

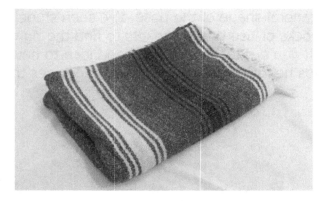

Blankets can be used in so many ways because you can fold or roll the blanket to fit your needs. If you decide to use a blanket during practice, choose a blanket that is easy to move. Large blankets may be bulky and difficult to manage. I use Mexican blankets. The Mexican blankets are usually pretty inexpensive and easy to find. This blanket is 74 inches long and 52 inches wide. It is just the right size to cover up during Savasana.

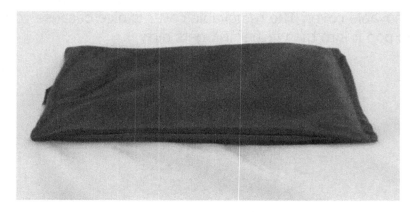

An eye pillow is a deluxe addition to the props. This pillow is filled with lavender and flaxseed. You can find eye pillows with different scents or unscented. The fabric has a silky texture which feels nice against the skin. The pillow is light but still has enough weight to feel pleasant when placed over the eyes. I use one during Savasana. They eye pillow completely blocks out the light and I enjoy the scent of lavender.

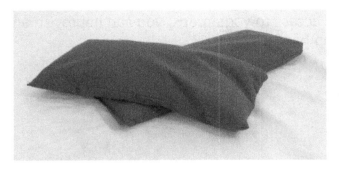

In addition to blocks, bolsters, and blankets, we have sandbags at our studio. These sandbags weigh about two pounds each. You can vary the amount of weight by the material you use to fill the bags and by the amount of material you add. The sandbags add gentle encouragement for the body to deepen into poses without using strength from the muscles.

When I was looking for sandbags for the studio, I was met with sticker shock. I was looking at buying one unfilled bag for $15. I wanted to have enough for 20 people to have at least one bag. Do the math. That adds up to a big investment. And that is just for the bag without the filling.

I decided to make my own sandbags. I borrowed a sewing machine from my daughter. I went to a big box store that sold fabric and purchased heavy duty outdoor fabric. After the fabric was cut into pieces that would make a nice rectangle bag, I sewed the fabric so that there was an opening left at the top of the bag. I purchased a big 50 pound bag of rice and used that as the filling. In no time I had 20 sandbags at a tiny fraction of what I would have paid for commercial sandbags.

Buying props can become very expensive. Just one bolster can cost $50 or more. Buying a single yoga block can run you as much as $24. A blanket from one of my favorite producers of yoga mats and accessories is $44. Yoga is not about acquiring stuff so stay within your budget. If you do not have access to yoga props, you can improvise and use what is on hand.

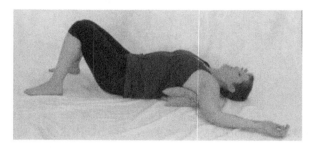

A bolster can be replaced by firm pillows. Grab a pillow from your couch or the bed for your home practice. The pillow in the picture came right from my couch. Choose a pillow that is soft enough for your comfort but sturdy enough to give your body the support required.

If you are feeling adventurous and crafty, You could make your make your own bolster without too much trouble. This is a no sew project that requires very little crafting skill. You will need a piece of fabric, a blanket or towel, and ribbon or rubber bands.

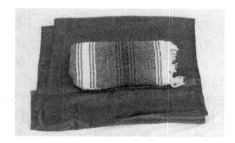

The fabric I used was purchased from a big box store

for $3/yard. I plan to use it later to make eye pillows. Make sure your fabric is big enough to cover the blanket or towel you will be using. If you buy one yard of fabric, it should be more than enough fabric to make one homemade bolster.

Roll the blanket or towel into the shape you want for your bolster. Wrap the fabric around the blanket or towel as tightly as you can. Use a couple of rubber bands on the ends of the fabric to secure it in place. Ribbon around the rubber bands would add a pretty and decorative touch to the bolster.

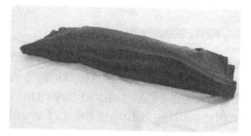 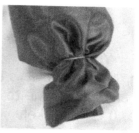

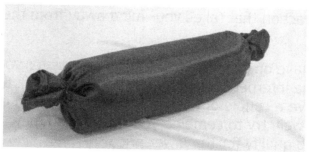

This is the end product for my homemade bolster. If you wanted to make the bolster larger, you could use additional blankets or towels until you have the size that is perfect for your practice. The whole thing comes apart as soon as you remove the rubber bands or ribbons if you want to use the items for a different purpose.

Some people have used books in place of blocks. I am not convinced that is the safest way to go. Blocks are often used under the seat to lift the hips higher to relieve pressure for the low body. A book seems a little too unstable. Buy yoga blocks. I hear they can be purchased at very reasonable prices from discount stores.

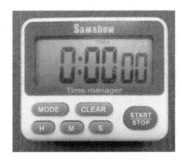

You will need some sort of timer to keep track of how long the pose is. This timer allows me to set the time I want and also allows me to see how far I have gone over the set time. It is very likely your phone has a timer on it. I would discourage using your phone. Just the site of the phone may be a distraction that takes your mind away from the practice.

I have one last tip about buying props for yoga. Search the internet for companies that sell in bulk to studios. If you have a couple of friends who are interested in buying props as well, try to combine your order. You may have enough to qualify for the lower price.

Props have the power to greatly enhance your Yin yoga practice. Use them thoughtfully each time you enter a pose.

CENTERING

Before bringing the body into Yin poses, spend some time centering. Find a seat on the mat that allows you to sit upright and feel reasonably comfortable. I like to sit in firm pose (kneeling with the hips on the heels) with a block or two under the hips. I see other students sitting in easy pose (shins are crossed). I see some students sitting on a folded blanket with the legs straight out in front of them. Most bodies sit with greater ease when the knees are lower than the hips. The exact shape is not important. What is important is finding a space with enough effortlessness that your mind is able to quiet.

Sitting up tall allows the spine to stack and the body to have space to breathe. Begin centering by bringing all of the attention to the breath. Know the very moment the inhale begins. Follow the breath as it moves through the body. Begin to notice physical changes in response to the breath. Watch the way the shoulders lift, the ribs expand, and the belly presses out on the inhale. Hold the breath for a moment at the top of the breath. Try to fully experience the inhale breath.

Give just as much attention to the exhale breath. Feel the way the exhale breath is a little warmer as it exits from the nose. Acknowledge the way the physical body begins to soften and release on the breath out. Spend a moment in stillness at the bottom of the exhale breath. Fully experience the exhale breath.

The body seems to lift and energize on the inhale breath. On the exhale breath the body may settle down into its space. The pauses between the inhale and exhale allow for moments of quiet reflection.

The length of the inhale and exhale is not as significant as keeping the focus on the breath. The breath fullness may even change the longer you sit and center. The number of breaths may also decrease the longer you spend centering.

Prana is the Sanskrit word for "life force". Each time you breathe in you are breathing in life force. On a scientific level that life force is the oxygen your body needs to survive. On a yoga level you may think of your inhale as a way to breathe in energy that nourishes your body. The body may feel stronger and longer on the inhale. Feel all of the changes your inhale breath brings to your mind and body.

Each breath out is your body's way of flushing out gasses your body does not need like carbon dioxide. As you breathe out in your yoga practice, you might envision symbolically letting go of anything that is holding you back on a physical, emotional, or spiritual level. You can let go of physical tension with your exhale. You might imagine letting go of anything that is in the path of reaching a space of peace and calm. Notice the softness in the body after the exhale.

Centering allows the body to settle and quiet down and also allows the mind to settle and quiet. Giving the mind a task like watching the breath can help the brain let go of its constant stream of thoughts. The goal of centering is to bring the mind and body into a space of being present and being aware.

During centering you may wish to introduce a mantra to help you concentrate the mind into a single point of focus.

A mantra is a word or phrase that can be repeated over and over. You may repeat the mantra during centering, a few times during each Yin pose, or repeat the mantra in each Yin pose as often as each breath. The word or words you choose are up to you.

As you center the mind and body and focus on your breath, your mind becomes quiet and still. In that stillness a mantra may come to you. Without forcing yourself to create a mantra, see if something pops into your mind. Decide if this word or phrase will be productive to repeat during your centering or during your Yin practice.

You may find that your mantra comes to you right away on some days. There is no effort involved as the perfect word or phrase reveals itself. You know as soon as you think it that this is where you should focus today.

Some days it may feel like you are investing tremendous effort in searching the mind for a mantra without bringing you any closer to finding your mantra. Here are a few words that might inspire you to use as a mantra:

Stillness	Happiness	Trust
Strong	Contentment	Dream
Focused	Fulfilled	Greatness
Love	Abundance	Creativity
Peace	Gratitude	Believe
Acceptance	Grateful	Powerful
Success	Fearless	Bliss
Joy	Forgiveness	Let Go

Your mantra does not have to be a word that you recognize. Mantras can be associated with sounds that you repeat. There are seven seed mantras or sounds associated with the main seven chakras. If you would like to concentrate on opening a specific chakra during your practice, you might start by saying the seed mantra for that chakra. You can repeat the sound a few times until you feel the energy from that sound begin to resonate in your body. Come back to that sensation as you notice the mind wandering.

The seed sounds for the chakras are:

The seed mantra for the first chakra known as the root chakra or Muladhara chakra is Lam.

The seed mantra for the second chakra known as the sacral chakra or Svadhisthana chakra is Vam.

The seed mantra for the third chakra known as the solar plexus chakra or Manipura chakra is Ram.

The seed mantra for the fourth chakra known as the heart chakra or Anahata chakra is Yam.

The seed mantra for the fifth chakra known as the throat chakra or Vishuddha chakra is Ham.

The seed mantra for the sixth chakra known as the third eye chakra or Anja chakra is Om.

The seed mantra for the seventh chakra known as the crown chakra or Sahaswara chakra is the sound of silence.

Om may be used as a mantra on its own. Om is a sound that is said to allow you to feel as if you are in harmony with the universe. There are four different sounds when saying Om as a mantra. The beginning sound is "ah" and begins deep in the belly. The next sound is "oh" and moves up into the chest. The third sound is "mmm" which is felt as a vibration on the lips. The last sound is silence as you inhale. It is tradition for many people to begin each yoga practice or meditation session by repeating Om three times.

I feel very peaceful when repeating Om. There is a wonderful calming quality about the sounds as they resonate through the body. I have a favorite song by Soulfood called Om. Just listening to others repeat the mantra in unison brings me into a sense of tranquility. I like the song so much I sometimes play it while teaching Yang style yoga classes.

The concepts introduced in centering can be applied during Yin poses. As the mind begins to wander in the poses, remind yourself to come back to the breath or repeat your mantra. The breath or a mantra may help keep you present throughout the practice.

FINDING YOUR YIN POSE

Yin is all about allowing the practitioner to make adjustments and changes to each pose to come into a space where he or she can feel sensation in the body but also feel content enough to be still. There is a balance between the intensity and comfort of the pose. Only the student can say exactly where that space is. In order to guide yourself or another to that sweet spot, there are many variations for each pose. The body can be moved slightly or supported by a prop to find the perfect shape to experience a change in the body.

There is more than one way to enter and exit a pose. I offer suggestions for each pose but you may decide to set up a pose differently. Remember that your practice is your practice. As you spend more time exploring Yin poses, you may decide to use props in new ways that are perfect for your body. Trust your body as you practice.

Many people have become numb to their physical body. A person can be so detached from the body that they do not even realize when there is a problem. It is especially important in Yin poses to physically experience the pose. Use the information from the body to make adjustments in the pose.

I have decided to arrange the description of the Yin poses in this section in alphabetical order. I hope that allows you to find poses quickly when you are putting a class together as a teacher or looking for inspiration as a student.

Ankle Stretch

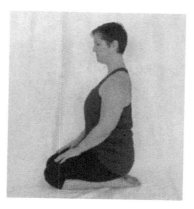

Just as the name implies this pose targets the ankles. Start by coming to the hands and knees in Table Top. The tops of the feet are on the mat. Begin to bring the hips back to sit on the heels. Check in with how your body feels in the ankles and the knees. If this is enough sensation, stop right here.

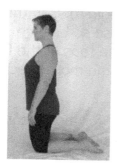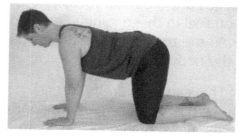

If you are feeling too much discomfort in the ankles or the knees, stand on the knees for a few moments. You could also come back to table top to take a break from the pose. Return to Ankle Pose when your body is ready.

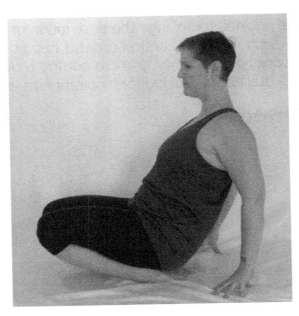

The standard ankle stretch may not be enough on some days. You may decide to lift the knees from the mat and lean back on your hands to deepen the sensation of the pose. Shift the weight from the center of the body toward the heels. The hands are there to offer support but you could lift the hands from the mat to balance.

After you have found the shape of the pose that is right for you. Come into stillness and begin to scan the body. The ankles are the main focus of the pose so begin exploring how you feel in these joints. Feel into the tops of the feet and even the toes. Feel the ankles become more spacious. Allow the body to settle.

This can be a pretty intense pose for most people. I tend to hold Ankle Stretch for a shorter time than most other Yin poses. As with all poses, if there is pain, exit the pose.

To come out of the pose, bring the hands to the mat and make your way back into Table Top. Spend some time in stillness as you absorb the effects of the pose.

Props for the pose:

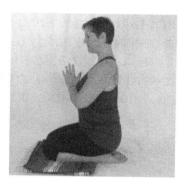

Place a blanket under the knees if the knees are tender.

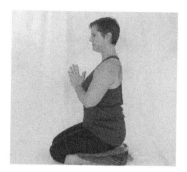

A blanket can be placed between the calves and hamstrings for tight knees.

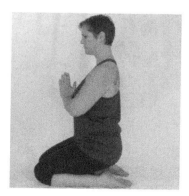

Sit on a block or bolster if there is too much pressure in the ankles, knees, or hips.

Variations:

Add a wrist stretch to the pose. Bring the palms to heart center and press the heels of the hands toward the floor. You could also point the fingers toward the floor and pull the heels of the hands toward the chin. To stretch the wrists in the opposite direction, bring the backs of the hands to press on the ribs.

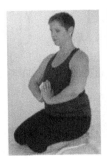 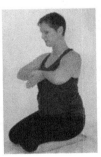 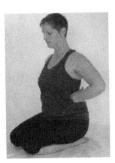

Bananasana

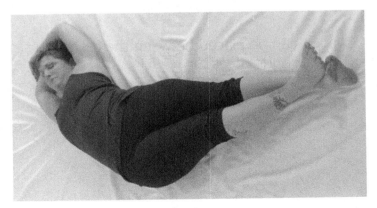

This pose helps to lengthen the side lines of the body while bringing a gentle curve to the spine. Lie flat on the mat. Keep the hips firm on the mat while walking the feet as far as possible to the left. Begin to walk the shoulders to the left while keeping the hips stable. Stop right here if you feel a deep stretch. For more sensation in the pose cross the right ankle over the left and reach the arms overhead.

This pose allows for a deep stretch on the side body. Begin to explore how your body reacts to the pose. Start at the toes and mindfully scan your way up the body. Do you feel sensation on the side of the ankle or leg? Notice if you feel a pull or tug around the hip or low back. Allow the upper side body to soften as you explore the upper arm and all the way to the fingertips. Let your body surrender to the opening.

Come out of the pose by releasing the arms and uncrossing the ankles. Walk the shoulders and feet back to center. Bring the spine back into alignment. Pause for a few breaths in stillness before bringing the body into the pose on the other side.

Bending Branch

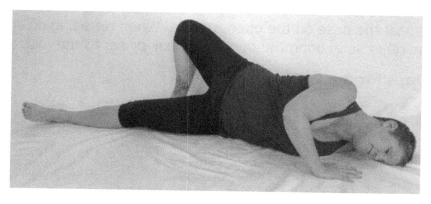

Begin the pose by lying flat on the stomach with the arms wide. The body will look like the letter "T" with the arms outstretched and the palms facing down. Bring the left hand under the shoulder. Bend the left knee so the toes point to the sky. Begin to roll to the right side of the body. The left foot will come to the ground behind the body with the knee pointing up. The hips and shoulders may stack on top of each other. Roll into a place that allows the right shoulder to open.

This pose is all about opening your shoulder. You can adjust the intensity by leaning back to feel more sensation. You could even bend both knees so the knees point toward the sky if that is the right place for your body to open. If the sensation goes beyond discomfort, bring the front of your body closer to your mat.

Once you are in the general shape of the pose, become still. Allow the muscles to loosen up and the connective tissue to stress. Observe how you feel in your shoulder. Scan for any tightness or muscular action in the shoulder and neck. Soften deeper into the pose as time moves on.

To release the pose roll back onto the belly. Bring the arms to rest beside the body with fingers pointing toward the toes and palms up. Rest the cheek or ear on the mat. Spend some time in stillness or do a counter pose here. Repeat the pose on the opposite side. When releasing on the other side, bring the opposite cheek or ear to the mat.

Props for the Pose:

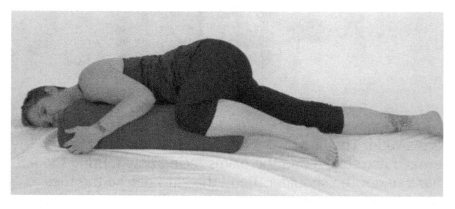

Use a bolster to support the chest or belly. If the pose is

too much for the shoulder, rest part of the chest, belly, and knee on the bolster.

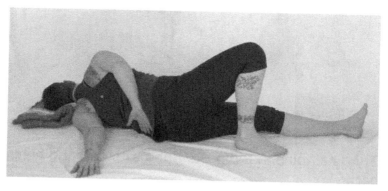

   To support the neck bring a blanket or block under the head.

Variations:

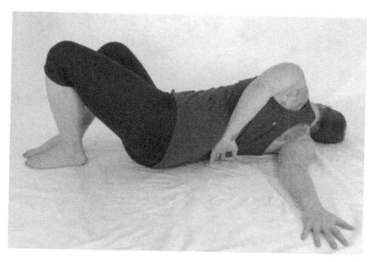

   If you want to increase the twist in the spine and apply more pressure to the shoulder, point both knees toward the sky. Begin to roll the top shoulder back toward the floor until you have reached the appropriate space for your body.

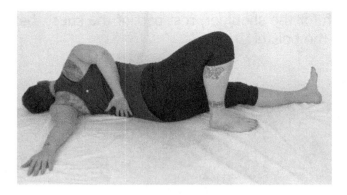

Try a half bind in the pose. Bring the top hand behind the back.

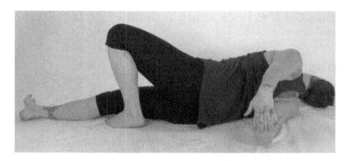

If the shoulders are very open, try interlacing the fingers behind the back.

Supported Bridge

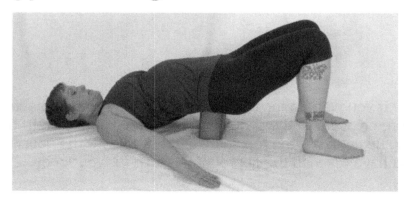

Supported Bridge pose uses a block to hold up the

spine while in a backbend. Start by lying flat on the mat with the knees bent and the feet flat on the floor. Press down through the feet and shoulders enough to lift the hips to a sufficient height to allow a prop to come under the sacrum. A block or a bolster can be used under the low back to support the spine in this bridge pose. I like to use blocks because the blocks are light and easy to move. Some may find the edges of the blocks too hard or firm. The bolster will give a little softer support. Arms can rest on the sides with the palms facing up.

Because the back is supported by a block or bolster, it may be easier to let go of muscular engagement in this Bridge pose. Think about the gentle bend in the back. Allow the shoulders to soften on the mat. Scan the spine to let go of any muscles that may be tight. Soften the buttocks and low back. Begin to observe sensations on the front of the body. Let the belly feel soft. Allow the chest to open and the heart to shine out.

To come out of the pose lift the hips enough to remove the prop and allow the hips to slowly return to the mat. Take a moment to lie flat on the mat with the knees stacked over the ankles.

Props for the pose:

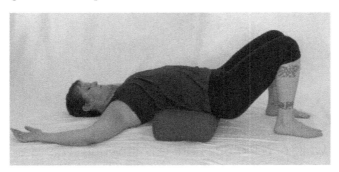

A block or bolster is placed under the sacrum to support the body.

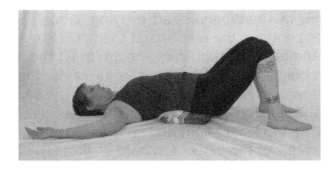

Use a blanket under the sacrum for less of a backbend.

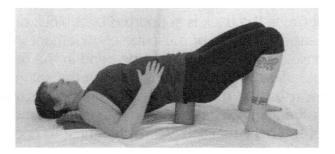

Try a blanket under the shoulders for softness under the upper back.

Variations:

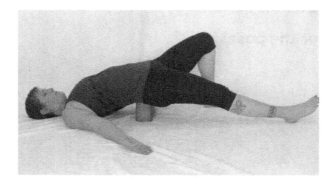

Begin to walk one leg out until it is straight. This is a wonderful stretch for the hip flexors. After some time bring the leg back to its original position and walk out the opposite leg

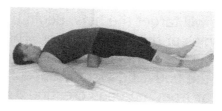

Walk both legs out so that they are both straight at the same time.

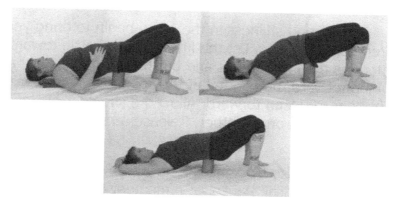

Change the position of the arms. Hands can be on the belly to connect with the breath and place less stress on the shoulders. Arms could be at cactus or reaching overhead to feel a different sensation for the shoulders.

Butterfly

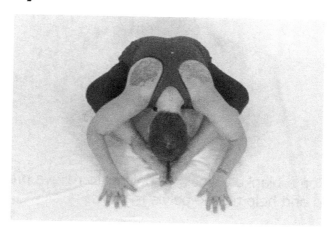

This pose will target the hips. Begin by sitting on the mat. Bring the soles of the feet together. There is a different sensation in the hips and inner thighs depending how close the heels are to the body. I generally encourage students to bring the heels far from the body creating a big diamond shape. If this is enough sensation then stop here. Folding forward may intensify the stress in the hips and allow the spine to bend.

As you find stillness in the pose, begin to bring your awareness to the hips. Let the knees gently settle toward the floor as the inner thighs and buttocks soften. If you are rounding forward, be mindful of the spine. Feel space in the low back as you lean forward. Allow the shoulder blades to soften away from one another. Release tension in the neck and scalp.

Exit the pose by using the hands to walk the upper body back to vertical. Pause for a moment once the spine is stacked. Release the legs and hips and pause for a few breaths.

Props for the pose:

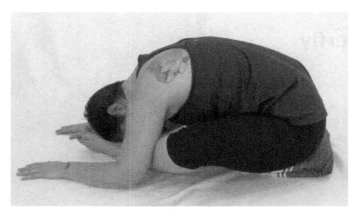

Sit on a blanket, block, or bolster to relieve pressure in the hips and help tilt the pelvis forward.

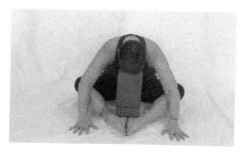

Use a block or stack of blocks under the forehead to support a tender neck when rounding forward.

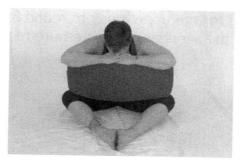

Place a bolster on its side across the knees to support the upper body. The bonus effect of using the bolster in this way is the weight of the bolster pressing on the knees. This pressure may help the hips stretch into a deeper position.

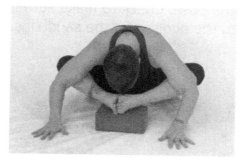

Try a block under the feet for a different sensation in the hips.

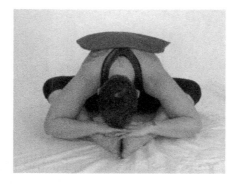

A sandbag placed on the upper back will offer gentle encouragement for the upper body to round forward a bit more. Remove the sandbag if the pressure feels too intense.

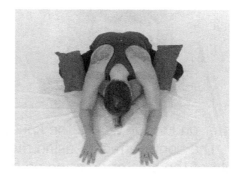

Sandbags can be placed on the knees or inner thighs to gently deepen the pose. Check to make sure there is not too much strain with the addition of the sandbags.

Variations:

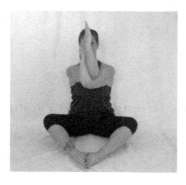

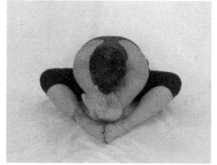

Open the shoulders by adding Eagle arms. For Eagle arms you will bring the right arm under the left. Hook the arms at the elbows. The thumbs will be toward your face. The backs of the hands will touch or the palms can come together. You can keep the upper body upright or fold forward with Eagle arms. When folding forward, allow the elbows and hands to gently fall toward the floor with minimal effort. Be sure to balance the same amount of time in Eagle on the other side with the left arm under.

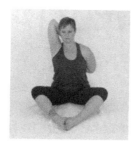 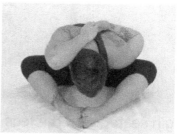

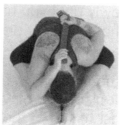

Open the shoulders with Gomukhasana arms. Gomukhasana arms start by sweeping the right arm high and bending the elbow so that the right hand rests on the back. The left arm reaches out to the left and then up the back. The hands may connect. If the hands do not connect, use a strap to bridge the gap. Leaning forward may change the sensation for the shoulders.

Balance the work in the shoulders by doing the same bind on the other side with the left hand resting on the back and the right arm coming out wide then reaching up the back to connect with the left hand. Use a timer to make sure you give equal amounts of time on each side.

Caterpillar

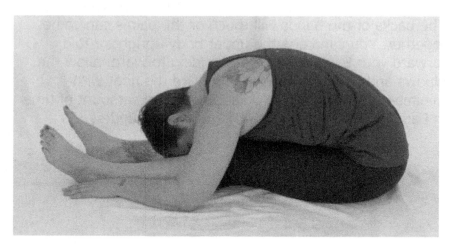

Begin seated with the legs straight. Start to fold the upper body toward the floor as the hands walk down the legs. Round forward slowly until you have reached the perfect spot for you. The head may drop toward the floor.

When you have found the shape you wish to hold, start to take notice of the area which feels the most stress from the pose. The first place you may feel sensation is the hamstrings. Do your best to soften the back of the legs and the tops of the legs. Notice if you are flexing your ankles or reaching for your toes. Let go of strength in the low body. If you are rounding forward notice the feelings along your spine. Allow the low back to broaden and the upper back to release.

When you are ready to leave the posture, walk the hands up the legs until the spine is stacked. Sit for a few breaths in stillness with the spine stacked before moving the legs.

Props for the pose:

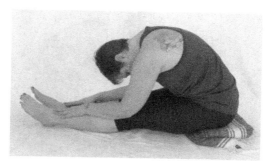

Sit on a blanket to elevate the hips and help tilt the pelvis forward.

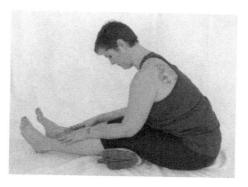

A rolled blanket can go under the knees to provide a slight break in the back line of the body for tight hamstrings.

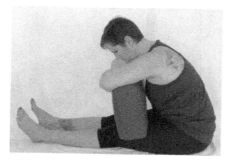

Use a bolster tilted on its side to support the upper

body. The arms will drape over the bolster and the chin or forehead can rest on the side of the bolster.

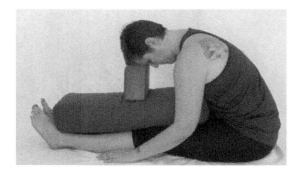

A bolster can be placed in line with the legs to support the upper body as you lean forward. Blocks can be used along with the bolster to provide a place for the head to rest.

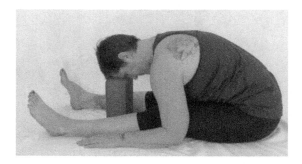

A stack of blocks can be used under the forehead to support the neck as the head drops toward the mat.

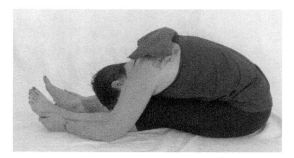

A sandbag can be placed on the upper shoulders or

along the spine to gently encourage a deeper fold.

Variations:

If you or your student has a lot of mobility, separate the feet wide enough to allow the head to come all the way to the floor.

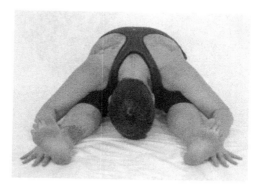

Dangle

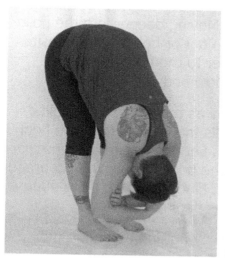 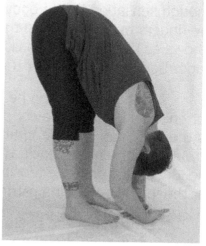

To begin Dangle Pose stand in Mountain Pose. Place the feet about hip width apart. Begin to walk the hands down the legs to come into a fold. The knees may be bent or straight.

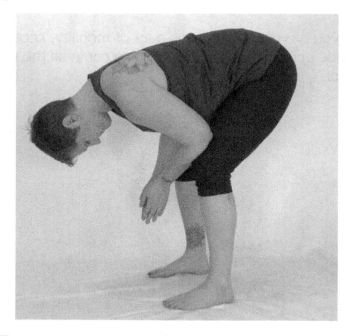

Forearms may rest on the upper thighs if this brings enough sensation to the body. Moving deeper into the pose the fingers may fall toward the floor or hold on to opposite elbows as the head comes closer to the floor. Allow the upper body to dangle over the low body.

The head will hang heavy as the neck and shoulders soften. Feel the way gravity pulls the head toward the floor as the neck and spine lengthen. Let go of as much muscular strength in the upper back as the body will allow. Encourage the low back to release tension. Find the appropriate edge for the legs. Feel the hamstrings begin to soften.

Come out of the posture by putting a bend in the knees and walking the hands up the legs. Lift out of the pose slowly to avoid feeling very dizzy upon standing. Be still for a moment once the body is upright.

Props for the pose:

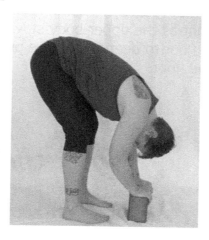

A block or a stack of blocks can be used under the hands for support.

Dragon

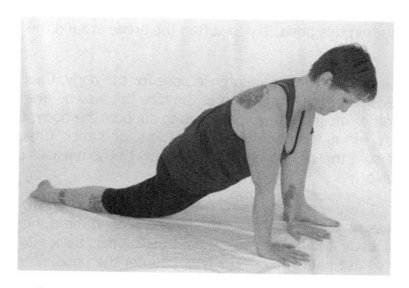

Start in Table Top. Bring the right foot to the outside

of the right hand. Bring the foot a little closer to the right side of the mat if that feels more comfortable. The arms may remain straight as the upper body stays lifted or bring the elbows to the floor to deepen into the pose. The head may tilt toward the floor.

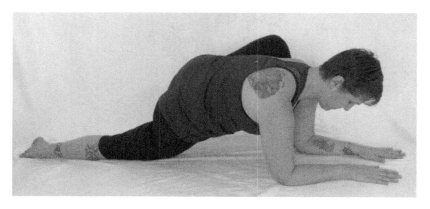

Ease into the hips and find stillness. Begin to notice the sensations from the hip connected to the front leg. How does this differ from the sensations of the hip connected to the back leg? Find the balance of releasing muscular strength in this pose. Try to soften the areas around the hips.

Dragon can be an intense pose for the body. Check for tension in the target area of the hips but also be aware that other muscles may tighten up to support the body. Be sure to soften the upper back, shoulders, and neck. Check to make sure there is no tension in the jaw or the muscles of the face.

Exit the pose by coming back to Table Top. In the stillness of Table Top notice the feeling around the right side of the body and the left side. Feel free to press back into Child's Pose until you are ready to counter the pose.

Hold for the same amount of time on the left side.

Props for the pose:

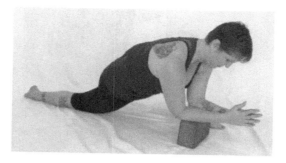

Rest the elbows on a block or a bolster to keep the upper body lifted a little higher. Remember that you can adjust the block height by turning the block on its side.

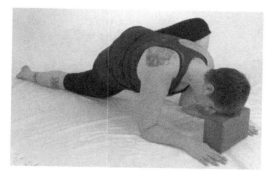

Bring a block under the forehead to support the head and neck.

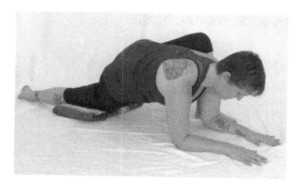

The bent knee that is touching the mat can rest on a blanket to offer comfort to a sensitive knee.

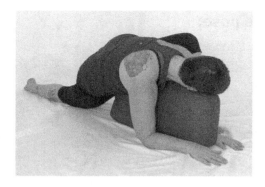

A bolster can be placed under the chest to support the upper body.

Variations:

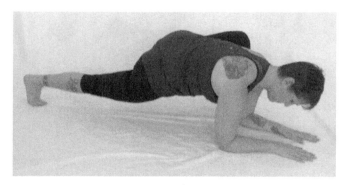

Fire Breathing Dragon is achieved by lifting the back knee from the floor. Be mindful of balancing the effort of the back leg with softening the hips.

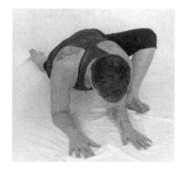

The Winged Dragon appears when the front knee falls

toward the outer edge of the mat. The inner edge of the foot may peel away from the floor. Point the toes in the direction of the knee to avoid stressing the knee. This is a deep variation of the pose so be mindful that you are keeping the stress to a safe level.

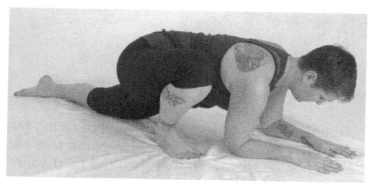

Try the Over Stepping Dragon by walking the front foot back until the knee is in front of the ankle. The heel may lift a bit from the floor. This is great for stretching the Achilles.

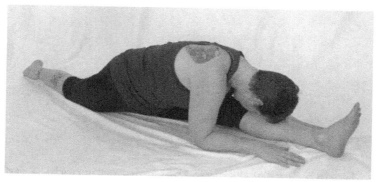

Dragon Splits is a variation of Dragon. Come into full splits by walking the front foot forward and the back foot back. Hands may rest on blocks as the upper body stays upright for stability. Bring the head to rest on the shin if the body has space.

Dragonfly

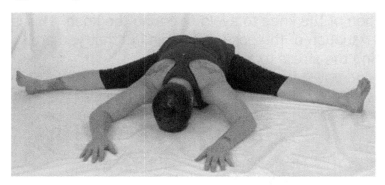

Turn your body on the mat so you are facing the long side of the mat. Turning to the long side of the mat allows the heels to rest on the mat rather than the hard floor. From a seated position separate the feet as wide as possible. Begin to walk the hands out in front of you as the pelvis tilts forward. Rest the upper body on the forearms or bring the chest to rest on the mat or floor.

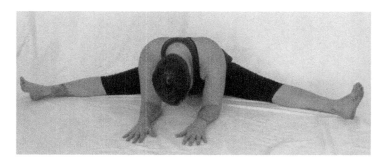

Find the general shape that suits your body. From that shape allow the body to become still and calm. Begin to scan for the space where you feel the greatest sensation. Notice if the ankles are flexed. Let the ankles and toes feel soft. Release tension from the back of the legs and the inner thighs. If there is pain in the low back, lift out of the pose until the pain ceases. Allow the upper body to soften as you lean forward. Release through the upper back and neck.

To leave the pose begin to use arm strength to walk the upper body to vertical. Pause once you are sitting up and feel the difference from leaning forward. Assist the legs by using the hands on the backs of the knees or thighs to guide the legs back together.

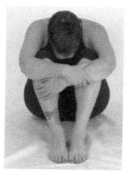 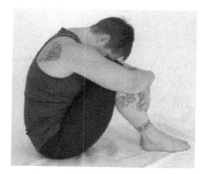

I often like to sit in an Upward Wind Removing pose with the arms wrapped around the knees for a few moments before straightening the legs or bringing movement to the body.

Props for the pose:

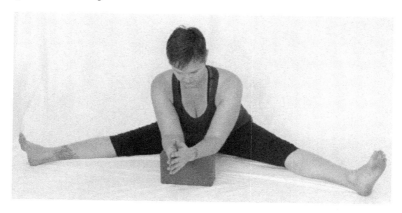

Use blocks or a stack of blocks under the forearms to keep the upper body lifted a little higher.

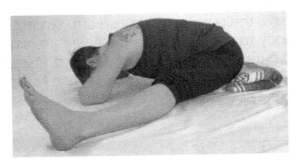

Sit on a folded blanket to lift the hips to ease pressure in the lower body. The folded blanket also encourages the pelvis to tilt forward.

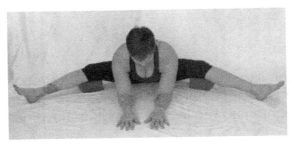

Use blocks or rolled blankets under the knees to relieve tight hamstrings.

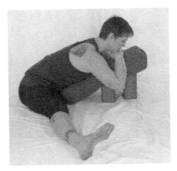

A bolster can slide under the chest to support the upper body. Blocks can be placed at different heights under the bolster to lift the bolster even higher. The blocks in this picture have been placed so that the first block is at the medium height and the next block is tilted to its highest elevation.

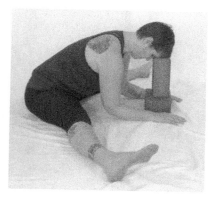

A block under the forehead can help support the neck.

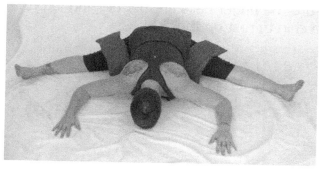

Sandbags can be placed on the top of each thigh to gently weight the legs and keep the body grounded.

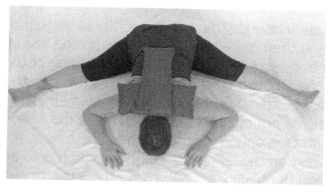

If the upper body is folded enough, sandbags can be placed on the upper shoulders to encourage the forward bend.

Variations:

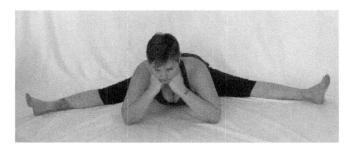

Rather than using props to keep the upper body lifted, try TV arms. Bend the elbows and make fists. When making fists be sure the finger nails are not digging into the palms. Allow the chin to rest on the fists.

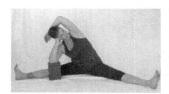 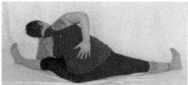

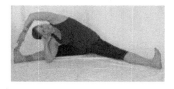

Include a lateral stretch in dragonfly to stretch the side body. Bring the right elbow to the floor on the inside of the right knee. A block or two can go on the inside of the knee to bring the elbow a little higher. Make a fist with the right hand (be sure to make the fist in such a way that the fingernails do not dig into the palm). Allow the head to rest on the fist. One option for the left hand is to stay at the waist or rest on the left thigh. Another option is to bring left arm behind the back for a half bind. The left arm can reach over head to deepen the stretch on the side body. Bring the arm to rest on top of the head. The last option for the left arm is to reach over head and softly touch the toes.

Remember to repeat on the other side for the same length of time.

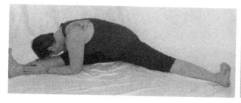 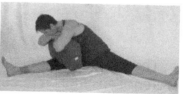

Folding directly over the leg may bring a different awareness to the low back and hamstrings. Shift the shoulders in the direction of the leg you are folding over and begin to bend toward that leg. A bolster can offer support if this brings too much of a strain in the low back or on the back of the leg. Balance the body by practicing on both sides.

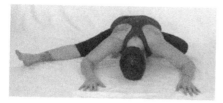 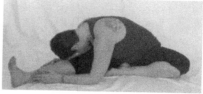

Come into Half Dragonfly from Dragonfly by bending the right knee bringing the right foot to the inside of the left thigh. From this position the upper body can lean forward through center. The upper body can also extend over the straight leg for a different experience. Be sure to practice on the right and left side for an equal amount of time.

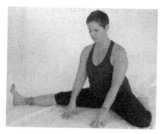 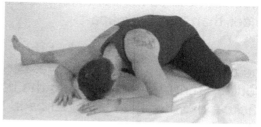

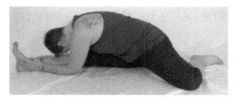 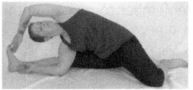

The right leg can bend in the opposite direction for a different sensation. Try bending the right knee so that the right heel comes toward the right hip. Bring the upper body through center or round over the left leg. Repeat with the left knee bent and the right leg straight.

Supported Fish

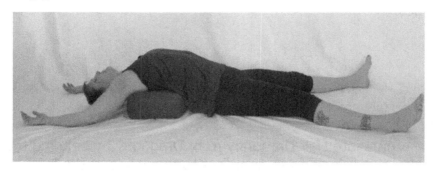

Position a bolster across the mat so when lying back the shoulders are supported. Slide the bolster under the shoulders in such a way that the top one or two inches of the shoulders are off the bolster. The arms can come out wide with the palms up. Extend the legs on the mat a little wider than hip width apart.

Allow the entire front of the body to soften. Feel that the chest is open and expansive. Let the collar bones widen. Notice if there is tension along the back in this supported backbend. Soften the shoulders and neck. Feel supported by the mat as muscles in the buttocks and the backs of the legs release.

When you are ready to change from the pose, roll to the side to release the bolster then roll back onto the mat. Lie flat on the back in stillness. If there is tension in the low back that prevents your legs from being straight while on the back, bend the knees and allow the knees to rest on each other while the feet are flat on the mat.

Props for the pose:

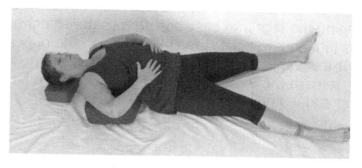

Place a block under the head to support the neck.

Variations:

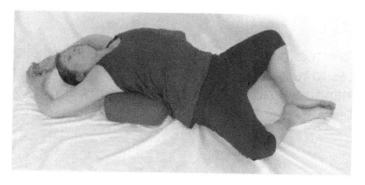

Change up the legs by taking Butterfly legs. Bring the soles of the feet together and let the knees fall open. Sandbags can be placed on the inner thighs or knees to deepen sensation in the hips.

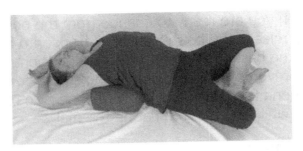

For a deeper sensation in the hips than Butterfly legs, try bringing the legs into easy pose (cross the shins) or bring the legs into square pose (the ankle rests on the opposite knee). If this variation causes too much stress on the knees or hips, release the legs. When taking this variation be sure to spend equal amounts of time on each side.

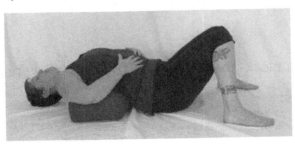

Soften the low back by bending the knees and allowing the knees to rest on each other. Place the feet on the mat wider than the hips. Place the hands on the belly to connect to the breath.

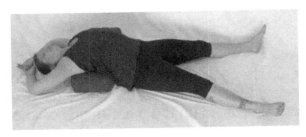

Change up the arms by bringing the arms over head. The arms can be straight with the backs of the hands on the floor or catch opposite elbows.

Frog

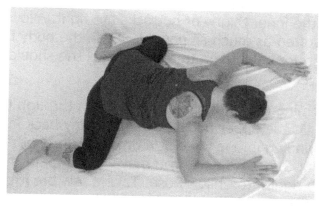

Your body takes up a lot of space on the floor in Frog so here are a few suggestions on how you might begin the pose. Turn on the mat so you are facing the long edge of the mat. Placing your knees on the mat in this position allows the knees to slide across the mat as the body deepens into the pose.

Rather than turning on your mat you could place a blanket across the mat. The blanket makes it easy to slide the knees apart as you are finding the appropriate shape of the pose. The blanket will support your knees if your knees slide off the mat.

Start in Table Top. Begin to separate the knees from one another as the body comes closer to the floor. The forearms come to the floor to help support the upper body. If the knees are separated very far apart, the chest may come down to the floor.

To feel more sensation the feet may separate so that the ankles are below the knees. To soften the pose a little, bring the feet closer together. Shifting the hips forward or backward may also change the intensity of the pose. Approach this pose mindfully and slowly until the body comes to a place where it feels safe to come into stillness.

Frog is a very powerful hip opener. Gravity helps your body open in this pose as the hips sink closer to the floor. Notice if the inner thighs or buttocks are tight. Allow the low body to soften as much as possible. Scan the body for other areas that are holding on to tension. Feel the shoulders and the neck let go.

Coming out of the pose press down through the hands to lift the upper body. Make your way back into Table Top by bringing in one knee at a time or bring both knees together at the same time. You may want to pause in Table Top or go right into Child's Pose. Take a few breaths to feel the difference in the inner thighs and hips.

Props for the pose:

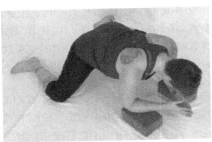

Bring blocks under the forearms to keep the upper body lifted a little higher.

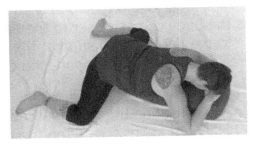

Use a bolster flat on the mat under the chest and belly to support the upper body. Use blocks under the bolster to lift the bolster to the desired height for sufficient support.

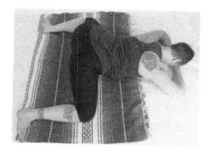

Use a blanket under the knees to allow the knees to slide apart from one another. The blanket may also provide softness for tender knees.

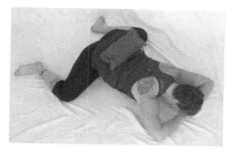

A sandbag can be placed on the low back to gently encourage the hips to open.

Variations:

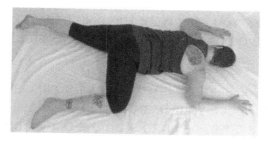

Try Half Frog for very tight hips and inner thighs. Start on the belly. Place one hand on top of the other and allow the forehead to rest on the hands. Bend the right knee so that the inner thigh is on the mat. Slide the knee toward the top of the mat for a deeper sensation and slide the knee toward the bottom of the mat for less sensation.

The arms may come out to the sides in a cactus position. If the neck allows, rest the right cheek on the mat. When the body is ready, come back to the beginning with both legs straight and the forehead resting on the hands. Repeat for the same length of time on the other side.

Legs Up the Wall

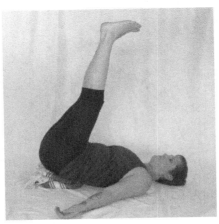

Begin Legs Up the Wall by lying on your mat. Bring your arms out wide. You may want the palms facing down toward the floor for a grounding effect. Lift the legs up toward the sky. The feet will stack on top of the hips.

This pose is said to be wonderful for circulation because your feet are above your heart. When you have found stillness in the pose, begin to scan the body from the toes to the hips. Soften the toes and ankles. Let the backs of the legs release tension. Feel the hips and buttocks soften. The back muscles can completely give in as the mat supports the back. Soften the front of the body. Let go of tension in the shoulders and the neck. Notice if your scalp feels tight. Settle completely into the pose.

When you are ready to release the pose, bring the feet to rest on the floor. Keep the knees bent and separate the feet wider than your hips. Let the knees rest against one another.

Props for the pose:

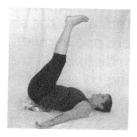

A blanket or block can be placed under the low back for support. The addition of this prop may allow you to use less strength to keep the legs in place.

Variations

Try changing the arms. The arms can come to a cactus with the elbows bent and the fingers pointing toward the top of the mat. Try another variations by allowing the hands to rest on the belly to connect to the breath.

Melting Heart

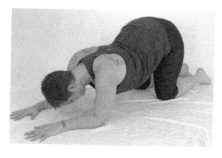

Come to a Table Top position. Bring the elbows under

the shoulders. Allow the heart to descend toward the floor. Keep the hips over the knees. Feel the upper back and shoulders curve as the chest opens and the collar bones widen. The head can drop toward the floor if the neck allows.

Notice where you feel the most sensation in your body. Let the neck soften. Allow the shoulders blades to smoothly squeeze toward one another. Have your mind travel the muscles from the base of the spine all the way up to your neck while letting go of all of the tension from your back.

Come out of the pose by bringing the hands under the shoulders and pressing back into Child's Pose. It might feel especially nice to allow the arms to rest beside the body with the fingers pointing toward the back of the mat. The forehead may rest on the mat or a block.

Props for the pose:

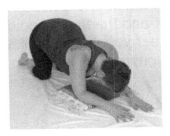

Use a blanket under the elbows for tender elbows.

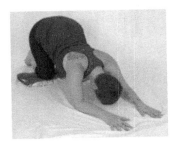

Place a blanket under the knees for tender knees.

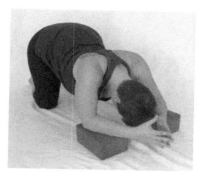

Place blocks under the forearms to allow more space for the heart to dip down toward the mat.

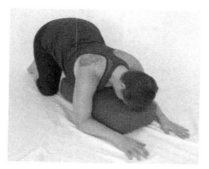

A bolster or blanket can go under the chest to support the upper body. Add blocks under the bolster to bring the bolster higher.

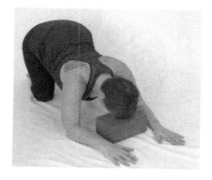

Use a block or blanket under the forehead to support the neck.

Variations:

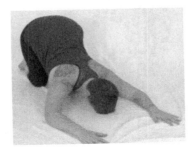

Change the arms by widening the space between the elbows.

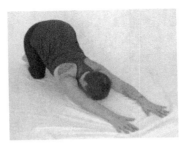

Another option to deepen the pose is reaching the fingertips forward so that the arms straighten allowing the chest to come toward the mat. The chest and forehead may rest on the mat.

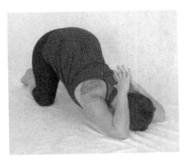

Bing the hands to prayer behind the neck for a nice stretch on the triceps.

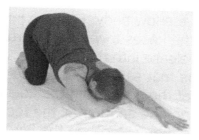

Try the Quarter Dog variation. From Melting heart bring the right forearm toward the body so it is parallel to the top of the mat. Extend the left arm forward. Allow the head to rest on the right forearm. Come back through Melting heart to switch to the opposite side.

Recline Butterfly

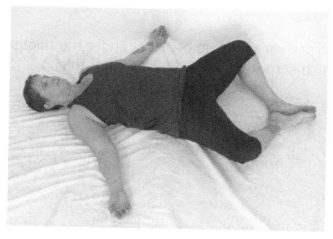

Lie down on the mat. From a reclined position, bring the soles of the feet to touch one another. Allow the knees to fall in opposite directions. Try adjusting the space between the heels and the body. Heels closer to the body may bring a different sensation to the inner thighs. Heels farther away from the body may change the way you feel in the hips.

As you find stillness in the pose begin to observe what

you are feeling in the low body. Feel the inner thighs open as gravity draws the knees toward the earth. Feel the hip sockets begin to release into the pose. Let go of any tension in your back as the mat supports your upper body.

To come out of the pose bring the knees together. The knees will rest upon one another as the feet are flat on the floor. Separate the feet wider than the hips.

Props for the pose:

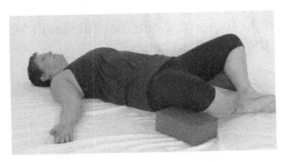

Try blocks or rolled up blankets under the thighs if there is too much sensation in the hips or inner thighs.

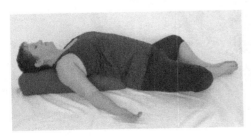 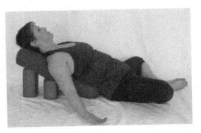

Use a bolster underneath the back. The height of the bolster can change by placing blocks under the bolster.

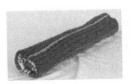 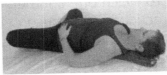 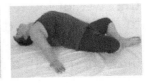

A rolled blanket or a block can be placed between the shoulders to lift the heart. The rolled blanket will feel softer than the block. The block may give you a higher lift and deeper sensation in the chest and back.

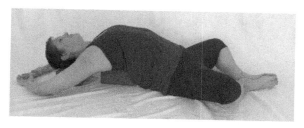

If there seems to be too much tension on the neck as the head tilts back, try placing a block under the head for support.

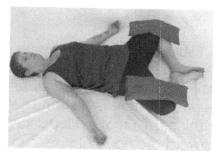

Sandbags can be placed on the inner thighs or knees to encourage the thighs and hips to open.

Variations:

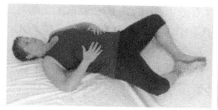
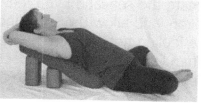

Change the position of the arms. The arms can be beside the body with the hands resting on the belly as you connect with breath. The arms can be wide resting on the mat with the palms up. Another option is to reach the arms overhead and catch opposite elbows.

Saddle

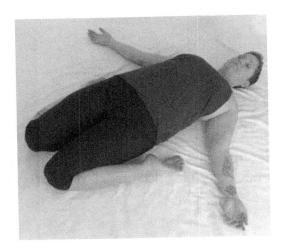

Begin in a Table Top. Bring the knees toward one another and separate the feet wider than the hips. Begin to bring the hips back to the mat as you sit upright. This can be the end of the pose if there is a strong sensation in the knees, ankles, or thighs. To move deeper begin to recline the upper body toward the floor. Elbows can come to the mat for support or bring the shoulders all the way onto the mat. Allow the arms to rest beside the body.

Listen to your body in this pose. Notice the tops of the feet and the ankles. Allow the knees to feel spacious. Locate the sensation you feel in the front of the thighs or hip flexors and allow the surrounding muscles to soften. If you are feeling tightness in the buttocks, let the tension soften. When leaning all the way back, be sure to notice how you feel in the back muscles. Release any strain in the low back and shoulders.

To come out from full Saddle, use the elbows to press into the mat to lift the upper body. Bring the hands to the mat and come back into Table Top. Child's Pose or Downward Facing Dog may feel good to the hip flexors and spine after Saddle.

Props for the Pose:

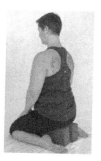

Sit on a block if the knees, ankles, or hips feel tight. If sitting on the block stay in an upright position and allow the ankles and knees to stretch.

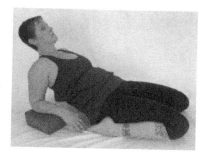

Use blocks under the forearms if you want a little support while leaning back. Leaning on blocks or a stack of blocks will keep the upper body lifted and may ease some of the sensation from the pose.

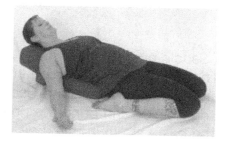

A bolster can be used under the back for support. Add a block under the bolster to lift it higher.

Variations:

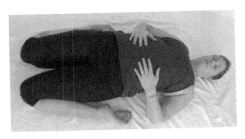

Rest the hands on the belly to connect to the ebb and flow of the breath.

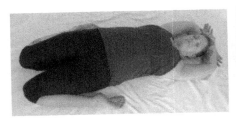 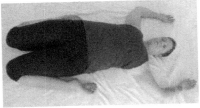

Bring the arms overhead if you are in full Saddle and want a little more sensation in the body.

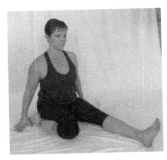

I prefer Half Saddle over Saddle when I am teaching and practicing. Try Half Saddle by starting in seated position with both feet forward and legs straight. Use the right hand to hold onto the right ankle and bring the right foot toward the right hip. If there is a strain in the knee, sit on a block or folded blanket. If there is stress in the ankle, squeeze a bit of blanket or a rolled up hand towel under the ankle. The pose can stop right here.

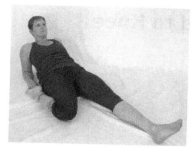

To feel a deeper sensation, begin to lean back. Let the forearms rest on the mat or blocks. Avoid leaning back on the hands as the wrists may become sore over time.

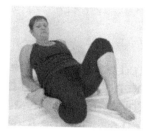

Try bending the straight leg to deepen sensation in the front of the thigh.

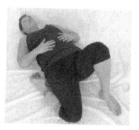 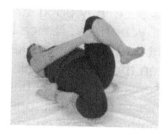

The shoulders may come all the way to the mat. If your body wants to go for an even deeper sensation, interlace fingers behind the thigh and pull the left knee to the chest. Find a space where you can soften through the shoulders, back, and legs. This variation can be very intense so be sure to be mindful and come out of the pose slowly. Repeat on the other side for the same amount of time.

Seated Head to Knee

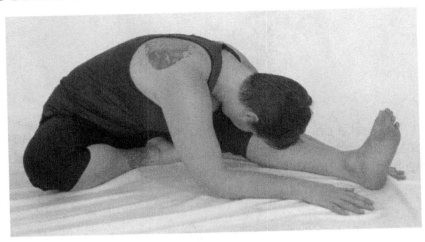

Begin in a seated position on the mat with both legs outstretched. Bend the right knee and bring the right foot to the inside of the left thigh. Begin to walk the upper body down the extended leg so that the forehead comes toward the knee. Feel the right knee fall to the floor as the hip begins to open.

This pose may bring strong sensation to more than one part of your body. Notice how you feel on the back of the straight leg. Feel the back leg muscles release into the pose. Soften the toes and ankle of the extended leg. Begin to detect sensations on the bent knee side of the low body. Let the inner thigh and hip open on the bent knee side. Release tightness in the buttocks. As you round forward try to allow the low back to broaden. Feel the shoulder blades soften and release stress.

Exit the pose by walking the upper body back to its upright position. Assist the bent knee by bringing the hand under the knee or thigh as the leg straightens. Repeat with the left knee bent and the right leg straight.

Props for the Pose:

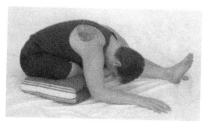

Use a blanket or a block under the bent knee to support the hip and inner thigh.

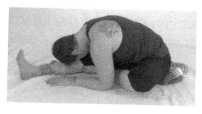

Sit on a blanket to lift the hips if the back line is tight.

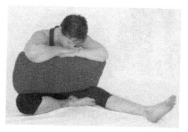

Use a bolster tilted on its side for a tight or tender low back. The bolster will sit on the legs as the upper body drapes over the bolster.

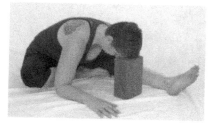

Place a block or tower of blocks under the forehead to support the neck.

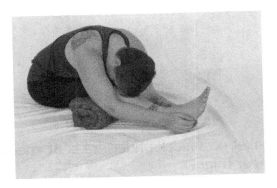

A rolled blanket can go under the knee of the straight leg for tight hamstrings.

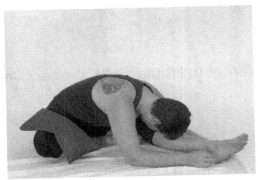

A sandbag can be placed on the knee or inner thigh of the bent leg to encourage a stronger stretch for the hip and inner thigh.

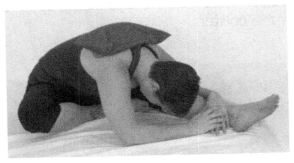

A sandbag may be placed on the upper back as the body leans over the extended leg to encourage a deeper fold.

Variations:

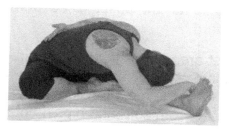

Add a twist to the pose by reaching the right hand toward the left foot. The right cheek may rest on the left shin. A half bind can be added by bringing the left arm behind the back. Repeat on the opposite side.

Shoelace

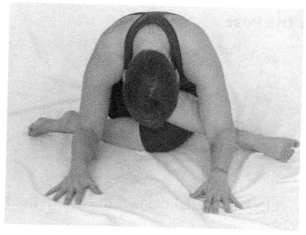

Start by sitting on the mat. Bend the right knee so that the knee points toward the top of the mat. The right heel may come toward the left hip. Bring the left leg on top of the right. The knees may rest on top of one another. This can be the pose right here. Stay upright if the hips feel very tight.

Sliding the feet away from the body may make

sensation in the hips more intense. Bringing the heels closer to the body may soften the pose. To deepen further begin to slowly lean forward.

The target area in this pose is the hips. Notice if there seems to be more sensation in one hip than the other. Focus on the site that feels the most tension. Allow that place to let go and release. From softened hips mentally scan out searching for more tightness or resistance. Let each place soften until you feel the body surrendering to the pose completely.

Come out of the pose by using the hands to press into the mat to lift the upper body. Support the legs by holding onto the foot and knee of the leg as it straightens. After sitting in stillness for a few moments, it may feel very nice to pedal out the legs. Repeat on the other side.

Props for the Pose:

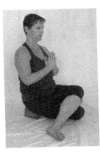 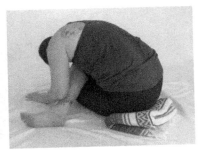

Sit on a block or folded blanket to elevate the hips if the hips are tight.

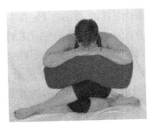

Use a bolster tilted on its side to support the upper body

in a fold. The bolster will rest on the legs while the upper body leans over the bolster.

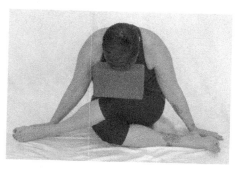

Stack a block or two under the forehead to support the head when leaning forward.

Variations:

Add a shoulder stretch by coming into Eagle arms or Gomukhasana arms.

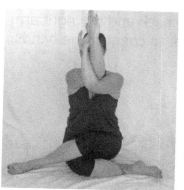 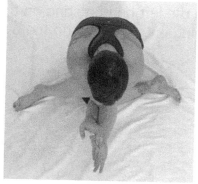

Open the shoulders by adding Eagle arms. For Eagle arms you will bring the right arm under the left. Hook the arms at the elbows. The thumbs will be toward your face. The backs of the hands will touch or the palms can come together. You can keep the upper body vertical or fold forward with Eagle arms. Be sure to balance the same amount of time on the other side with the left arm under the right.

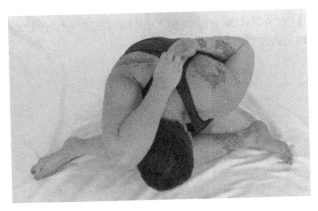

Open the shoulders with Gomukhasana arms. Gomukhasana arms start by sweeping the right arm high and bending the elbow so that the right hand rests on the back. The left arm reaches out to the left and then up the back. The hands may connect. If the hands do not connect, use a strap to bridge the gap. The upper body may lean forward for a different sensation in the pose. Balance the work in the shoulders by doing the same on the other side with the left hand resting on the back and the right arm coming out wide and up the back to connect the hands.

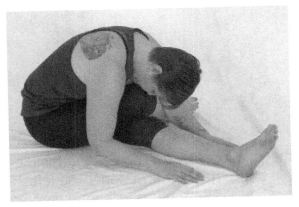

Find greater ease for the hips in Half Shoelace by straightening the bottom leg. Notice the difference in the hamstrings of the extended leg.

Sphinx

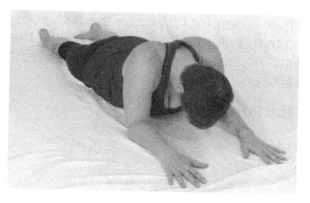

Lie on the belly. Bring elbows directly under the shoulders. The forearms and hands will rest on the mat. Allow the heart to melt toward the mat. The head may drop toward to floor if that does not stress the neck. There is a slight change in the feeling on the low back based on the position of the legs. The legs may be spaced wider than the hips so that the feet are toward the edge of the mat. My body feels more comfort in the low back with the feet wide.

Another option for the legs is to bring the toes to touch while the heels fall open. Notice how the back and hips feel with the toes close.

As the body finds stillness in the pose, feel the shoulders blades pull toward each other as the chest expands. Release tension in the neck and feel a nice stretch in the neck as the head drops toward the floor. Explore the upper, middle, and lower back for stress. Feel the low back broaden as the buttocks soften. Let the back side of the legs yield to the pose. Be aware of the front line of the body. Feel the support of the mat under the belly and tops of the legs.

Come out of the pose by brining the upper body to rest on the mat or press back to Child's pose. If you are bringing the body onto the mat, place one hand on top of the other and allow the forehead to rest on the back of the hands. Another option for resting on the belly is to bring the cheek to the mat, bring the arms to rest beside the body with the palms up, and bring the toes close together while the heels fall open.

Props for the Pose:

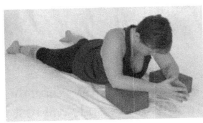

Use blocks under the forearms for a deeper opening of the upper back. This will lift the shoulders a bit higher and may feel like a deeper backbend.

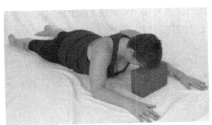

Place a block under the forehead to support the head and neck.

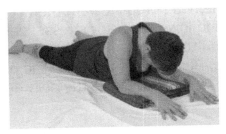

A folded blanket under the elbows can bring softness to the elbows.

Variations:

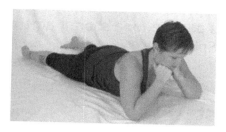

Find support for the neck and head without using a prop. Bend the elbows and make fists to create TV arms. Rest the chin on the fists.

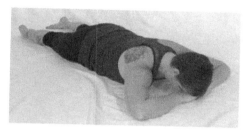

Lessen the pressure on the shoulders by bringing the upper body closer to the floor. Place one hand on top of the other at the top of the mat. Allow the forehead to rest on top of the hands.

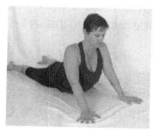

Deepen the backbend by coming into Seal. Press the palms into the mat and gently rotate the right hand to the right and the left hand to the left like little seal fins. Straighten the arms slowly as the back bend begins to deepen. If you would like a deeper backbend, walk the hands closer to the body. When you find the right place for the hands and the correct depth of the back bend, soften the body into the pose. Seal can be intense so you may want to hold this posture for a shorter amount of time than you would hold Sphinx.

Spinal Twist

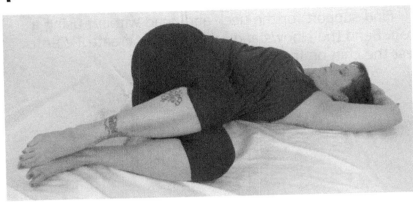

Begin Spinal Twist by lying on the back. Bring the feet flat to the mat and bend the knees. Shift the hips a few inches to the right. Bring the knees to the chest then allow the knees to fall over to the left. The right hip may stack on top of the left hip. The shoulders are resting gently on the mat. Arms can be wide with the palms down and shoulders resting on the mat.

Allow the spine to come into a gentle twist. Notice if you feel most of the sensation in the shoulders, back, or hips. Let tension begin to release from the site where you feel the most sensation. Let the release shine throughout your body. Feel the body give into the pose.

To come out of the pose bring the knees back to center and shift the hips to center. Take a moment to rest with the back supported by the mat and the spine aligned. Repeat on the other side for the same amount of time.

Props for the Pose:

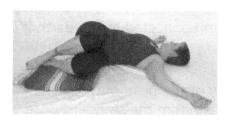

Use a block, blanket, or bolster under the knees if the knees do not come to the floor and the body would like support.

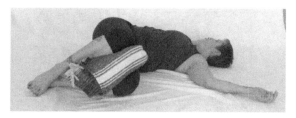

Use a block or blanket between the knees if there is an uncomfortable distance between the knees.

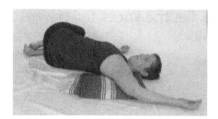

Place a blanket under the shoulder if it lifts to a place of discomfort during the twist.

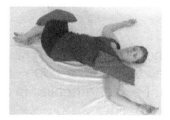

A sandbag on the thigh or knee of the upper leg can

encourage a deeper twist as the hips stack on top of one another. A sandbag on the shoulder or upper arm can help keep the shoulder connected to the earth if it begins to lift.

Variations:

The intensity of the pose may be changed by simply moving the knees. From the standard pose with the knees on the floor, bring the knees closer to the chest to feel an increase in sensation. Bring the knees away from the chest to lessen sensation.

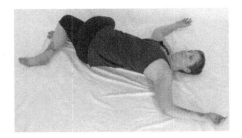

Try Twisted Roots variation. Eagle the legs by wrapping the right leg over the left. Wrap the foot around the leg if that is accessible. Let the knees fall toward the left. Repeat on the opposite side.

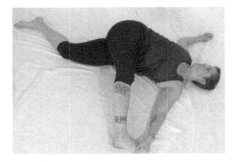

Try extending the top leg. If the knees are toward the left, use the left hand to hold the edge of the right foot. Extend the right leg. Feel lengthening in the extended leg. Repeat on the opposite side.

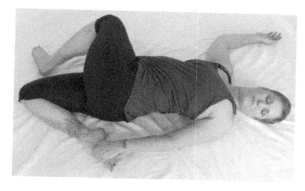

For a deep stretch in the hip flexors or quads, try binging the heel to the buttocks. If the knees are toward the left, Use the right hand to catch the left foot or toes. Pull the foot toward the body.

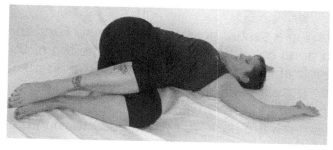

Try changing the arms. The arms can come to cactus by bending at the elbows.

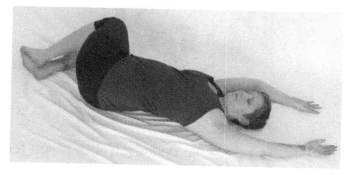

Reaching the arms overhead may change the sensation a bit more for the shoulders.

Square

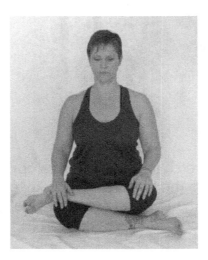

Start in a seated position on the mat. Bend the right knee and bring the right shin parallel to the top of the mat. Take the left ankle and place it on top of the right knee. This can be the pose if you feel a deep sensation in the hips. You can begin to round forward to deepen the sensation of the hips and stretch the back. Allow the body to round forward slowly and feel the intensity of the stretch.

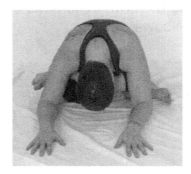

This pose is a deep hip opener. Notice if you feel greater sensation in the hip connected to the bottom leg or the top leg. Let your sensation scan begin at the point where you notice the most tension. Feel the muscles around that area begin to release. Soften the hips, buttocks, and leg muscles. If you are rounding forward give attention to the way the muscles around the spine are feeling. Let the low back feel spacious. Allow the shoulder blades to fall away from one another. Feel the stretch in the back of the neck if the head is bowing forward.

Release the pose by bringing the body to an upright position. Guide the left leg out of the pose by holding onto the foot and the knee as the leg straightens. Give a little support to the right leg by holding on under the knee or thigh as the leg straightens. After a few moments of stillness in the low body, you may want to pedal out the legs. Repeat on the opposite side.

Props for the Pose:

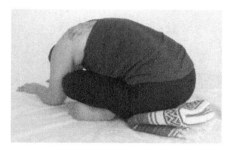

Sit on a block, folded blanket, or bolster to lift the hips and release tension for tight hips.

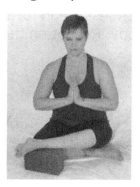

Use a block under the top ankle to relieve pressure in the hips. Move the top foot from the knee to rest on the block.

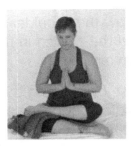

If the bony bump on your ankle brings discomfort to the leg it is resting on, place a blanket between the ankle and knee to soften.

Variations:

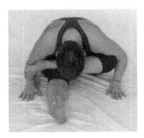

Half Square can be more accessible for tight hips. Start in a seated position on the mat. Extend the right leg. The left ankle will rest on top of the right thigh. Use a blanket under the ankle for softness. Lean forward as much as is appropriate for the body. Repeat on the opposite side.

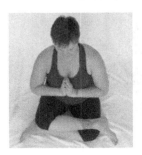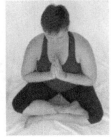

If sitting with the ankle on the knee is too intense for

the hips, try bringing the top of the foot to rest on the inside of the thigh or on top of your calf. Release even more by sitting in easy pose with the shins crossed.

Vary the arms to work into the shoulders.

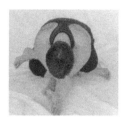

Open the shoulders by adding Eagle arms. For Eagle arms you will bring the right arm under the left. Hook the arms at the elbows. The thumbs will be toward your face. The backs of the hands will touch or the palms can come together. You can keep the upper body upright or fold forward with Eagle arms. Be sure to balance the same amount of time on the other side with the left arm under.

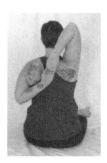

Open the shoulders with Gomukhasana arms. Gomukhasana arms start by sweeping the right arm high and bending the elbow so that the right hand rests on the back. The left arm reaches out to the left and then up the back. The hands may connect. If the hands do not connect, use a strap to bridge the gap. Balance the work in the shoulders by doing the same on the other side with the left hand resting on the back and the right arm coming out wide and up the back.

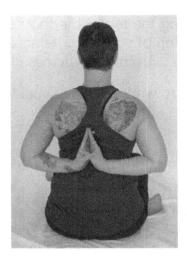

Open the shoulders in a different way by taking a different grip from behind. Try a reverse prayer with the hands. Bring the arms behind the back so that the palms touch.   Point the fingers up toward the sky. To lessen the sensation in the wrists, point the fingers toward the earth.

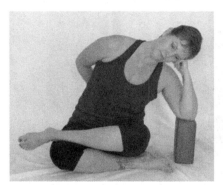 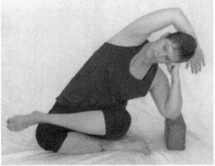

Stretch the sidelines of the body by coming into a lateral stretch. Place a block or stack of blocks on the side of the body. If the right leg is on the bottom, the blocks will go on the left side. Begin to lean toward the blocks and bring the elbow to rest on the blocks. The head will rest on the fist. The Right arm can come behind the back for a half bind or go overhead to stretch the upper arm. Allow the right arm to rest on top of the head when reaching overhead.

Swan

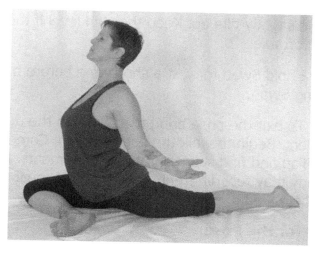

Begin Swan by coming into a Table Top position. Move the hands forward so they are in front of the shoulders. Bring the right knee behind the wrist toward the right edge of the mat. The right toes will slide forward toward the top edge of the mat. Walk the left toes toward the back of the mat. The right shin can be adjusted toward the top of the mat for a deeper opening. To soften a bit bring the foot closer to the body. Keep the upper body lifted for Swan. Palms may look toward the sky with the arms outstretched.

I find that the intensity increases in my body the longer I hold Swan. Be mindful about finding the general shape of Swan in the beginning of this pose. Notice if there is pain in the knee. If you are feeling pain, please adjust until the knee is no longer in pain. The target of this pose is the hips. Feel the muscles around the hip socket connected to the bent knee begin to release tension. Let the hip flexors on the side connected to the straight leg begin to soften.

Notice how the upper body feels in the lifted version of Swan. If comfortable the arms reach out with palms up creating a back bend. Let the upper back soften as the shoulder blades glide closer together. Feel into the neck as the chin slightly tilts up. Keep the chin level if the neck feels uncomfortable.

I hold Swan for just a short time before moving into Sleeping Swan.

To exit the pose bring the hands to the mat under the shoulders. Begin to walk the back toes up. Come back into Table Top and find stillness for a few moments. Notice how the body may feel different on one side. Repeat the pose on the other sided to open the opposite hip.

Props for the Pose:

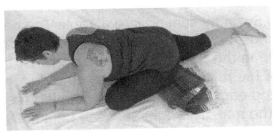

Use a block, blanket, or bolster under the hip or thigh on the side with the bent knee to give support to tight hips. If the hips are tight, spend extra time at the beginning of the pose to arrange a prop under the thigh until the body has sufficient support to find stillness in the pose.

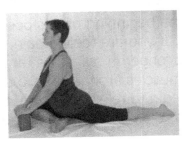

A block can be used under the hands to support the upper body while it is lifted in Swan.

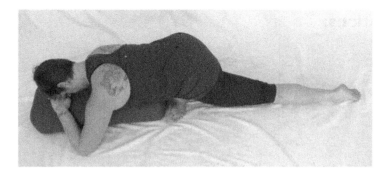

In Sleeping Swan a bolster can be used under the chest and belly to lift the upper body. Blocks may be placed under the bolster to lift the bolster to a height that best supports the body.

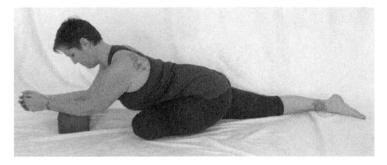

Blocks or a bolster can be used under the forearms to keep the upper body lifted in Sleeping Swan.

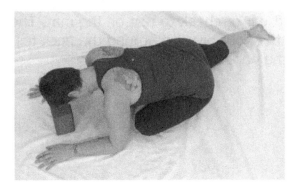

Place a block under the forehead to support the neck and head.

Variations:

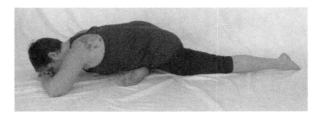

Sleeping Swan allows the upper body to fold forward. The upper body may lower so that the forearms and elbows are on the mat. The upper body may come all the way down to the mat. Place one hand on top of the other and allow the forehead to rest on the hands. Bring the upper body to a place that is comfortable enough to find stillness in the pose.

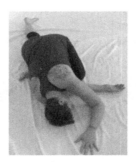

Try Sleeping Swan with a twist. Begin in Swan with the right knee bent. Thread the left arm under the chest and bring the left ear or cheek to rest on the mat. The right arm can rest on the floor or wrap around the back for a half bind. Repeat on the opposite side.

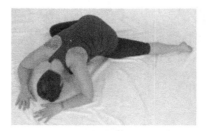

For a different sensation in the hips, try walking the

upper body toward the foot. Fold the upper body over the foot and allow the head to rest on the mat, back of the hands, or a block. Repeat on the opposite side.

Toe Squat

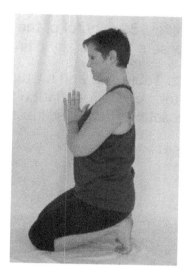

Start with the body in Table Top. Tuck the toes under. You may need to reach back and tuck the pinkie toe under if it is poking out. Begin to sit back on the heels.

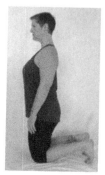

If it is too intense to sit on the heels, try standing on the knees. Come back to Table Top if this pose creates pain.

This pose may feel very intense for those who are on their feet all day or people who wear shoes that are not the most practical. Those with sensitive feet may want to enter this pose very slowly. Find the general shape the body wants to hold. Feel the spaces between the toes begin to open. Notice the bottoms of the feet. You may feel a stretch on the backs of the ankles. Be mindful of the stress in the knees. Adjust the pose if there is any pain.

Come back to Table Top and un-tuck the toes to exit the pose. Feel the tops of the feet flat on the mat and the toes still. Notice sensations during stillness.

Props for the Pose:

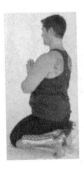

Place a blanket between the calves and hamstrings to support tight knees.

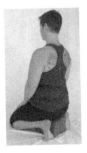

Sit on a block to keep the hips elevated and soften the intensity for the knees and toes.

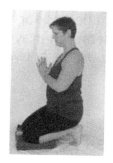

A blanket under the knees can soften the space for tender knees.

Variations:

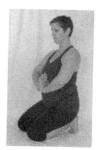 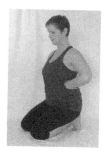

Add a wrist stretch to the pose. Bring the palms to heart center and press the heels of the hands toward the floor. To stretch the wrists in the opposite direction, bring the backs of the hands to press on the ribs.

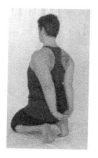 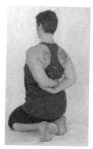 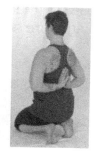

Add a shoulder opener by taking a grip behind the back. Simply interlace the fingers at the low back for a gentle stretch. Another option is to hold on to opposite elbows. Take prayer from behind for the deepest opening. The hands will come together in prayer behind the back so that the edges of the hands are between the shoulder blades.

Twisted Branches

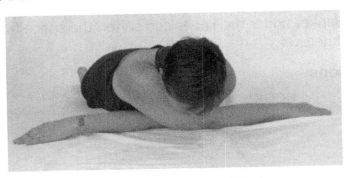

Start by lying on the belly. Bring the left hand under the shoulder and lift the upper body enough to slide the right arm under the chest. Reach the right fingertips toward the left. Bring the left arm in front of the right while reaching the fingers toward the right. The chin can rest on the left arm.

For a bit more pressure on the shoulders, tuck the toes under and use the feet to scoot your body slightly forward. This may bring more sensation to the shoulders.

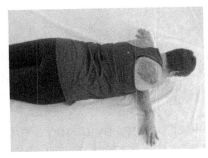

Feel the weight of the body open the right shoulder.

Soften the space under your right shoulder blade and upper shoulder. Let the neck yield to the pose. If you have both arms under the chest, try to find a balance so that both shoulders are opening and you feel the shoulder blades pulling away from one another.

Search for tension in the rest of the body. Allow the mid back and lower back to release into the pose. Mentally travel down the body and soften the buttocks, back of the legs, ankles, and toes.

To come out of the pose, bring the arms alongside the body with fingers pointing toward the toes and palms up. Rest the cheek or ear on the mat. Repeat the pose with the left arm under the chest first. When releasing on the opposite side, bring the opposite cheek or ear to the mat.

Props for the Pose:

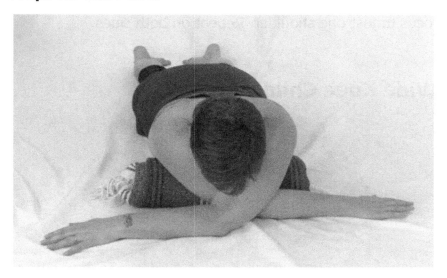

Bring a rolled up blanket under the chest. The blanket may lift the chest slightly to relieve stress in the shoulders.

Variations:

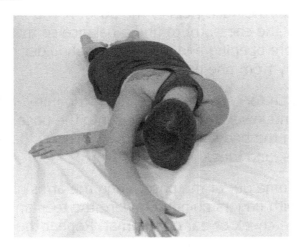

Try twisting just one branch. Bring only one arm under the chest. Allow the opposite arm to reach forward. This variation may allow you to deepen your awareness and focus to just one shoulder. Repeat on both sides.

Wide Knee Child's Pose

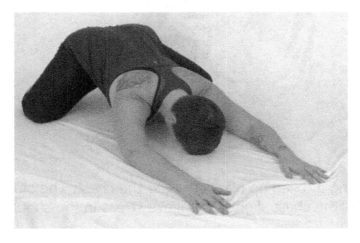

Begin in a Table Top. Bring the toes close together

and widen the knees. Begin to press the hips back to the heels. Reach the arms forward as the chest moves closer toward the mat. Allow the forehead to rest on the mat.

Search for sensation in the low body. Adjusting the space between the knees may change the way you feel in the pose. I like to separate the knees very wide as I feel a deeper opening in the hips in this position. When you have found the general shape that is right for the body, begin to notice the sensations in the ankles and knees. Soften into the hip area.

Observe the way you feel around the spine. With your chest on the mat and the arms extended, you may feel sensation in the upper back and neck. Feel the shoulders pulling toward one another. Allow the neck to soften.

Release the pose by bringing the hands under the shoulders. Lift the upper body so there is space for the knees to come together. You can press back into Child's pose or come to Table Top. Pause for a moment as you observe the sensations in your body.

Props for the Pose:

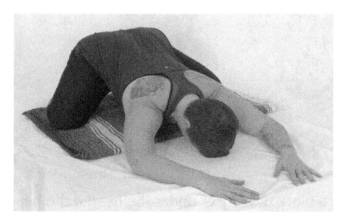

Bring a blanket under the knees. This will add softness under the knees and allow the knees to gently slide apart when entering the pose.

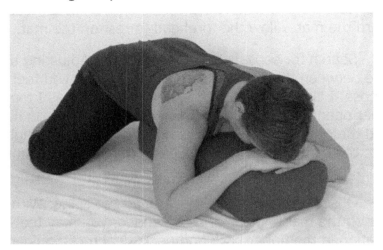

Place a bolster under the chest and belly for support as you lower the upper body. Use blocks under the bolster to lift the bolster higher. Keeping the upper body slightly lifted may lessen the sensation felt in the hips.

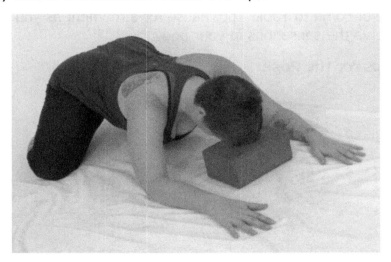

Use a block or blanket under the head if the head does not rest comfortably on the mat.

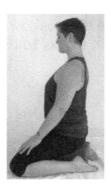

Lift the hips by sitting on a block to soften through the hips, knees, or ankles. The body can stay in the upright position on blocks.

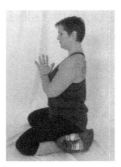

A blanket can be used between the calves and hamstrings to bring space for tight knees.

Variations:

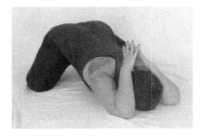

Stretch the triceps by bringing the palms to prayer. Bend

the elbows and bring the thumbs toward the back of the neck. Place the elbows on blocks to deepen the sensation.

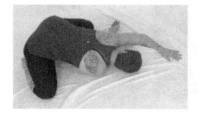 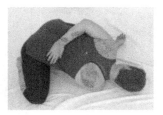

Add a twist to the pose. Lift the upper body and thread the right arm under the chest. Allow the right cheek to rest on the mat. Place a block or blanket under the head for support. The left arm can wrap around the back to add a half bind. Repeat on the opposite side.

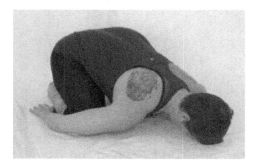

Arms can rest beside the body with the fingertips pointing back to soften through the shoulders.

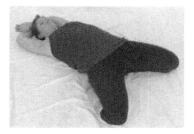

Try Reverse Wide Knee Child's Pose. From Wide Knee Child's Pose sit up on the heels. Begin to lean back onto the elbows or all the way back to the shoulders. Feel sensation in the ankles, knees, quadriceps, and hip flexors.

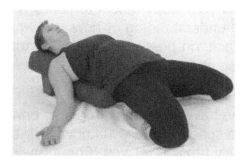

Use a bolster or a bolster in combination with blocks to provide support as you lean back in Reverse Wide Knee Child's Pose. Create more softness by using the bolster and blocks to lift the shoulders away from the floor.

Savasana

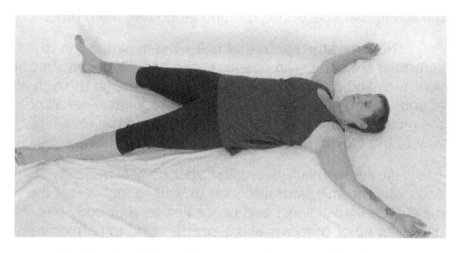

To find traditional Savasana lie on the back. Straighten the legs and separate the feet wider than the hips. Separate the arms wide with the palms facing up.

Now that you have made it to Savasana, you will use all of your knowledge about your body. During the Yin practice you have been getting intimate with your body. As you explore how your body reacts to poses, you gain knowledge and understanding of how and where you may hold tension. Each Yin pose offers an opportunity to learn how to find ease and comfort in different areas of your body. Put it all together in Savasana.

Once you have your body in place, bring your attention to the space where you know your body to hold the most physical tension for you. Common spaces that hold tension are the jaw, the neck, shoulders, low back, and buttocks. While these are the common places, you may hold tension in a different space. Listen to your body.

Begin to allow that space to soften. As you exhale the breath imagine that place in you beginning to yield. Each time you exhale the breath, that place responds by letting go. Repeat this process until you feel you have found success with this area. When you feel you have let go of all tension in that space, breathe and let go one more time.

Now that the space that holds the most tension is soft, take a mental scan of your entire body. You can start at your toes and mentally travel up the body. Let go through all of your joints. The big joints and the little joints. Feel all of the muscles give into Savasana as your mind travels all the way to the crown of your head.

At the moment you realize your body is perfectly still and peaceful, shift your attention to your thoughts. Let the mind settle into stillness and peace just as your body has done. Let go of concerns and allow the mind to harmonize with the tranquility of the moment.

You may want to revisit the way you began your practice when you centered. Come back to a breath that helps you settle. Recall your mantra if you created one. Slip into stillness of mind and body.

Props for the Pose:

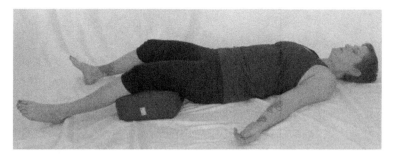

Use a bolster under the knees to soften the back line of the body.

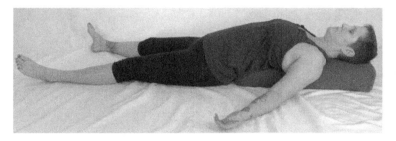

Place a bolster, block, or rolled up blanket in line with the spine to lift the chest and allow the chest to open.

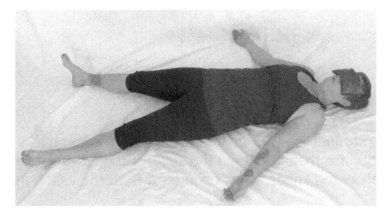

If you are distracted by lights during Savasana, cover

the eyes. You can use a simple hand towel to cover the eyes. Try a scented eye pillow for a luxurious Savasana.

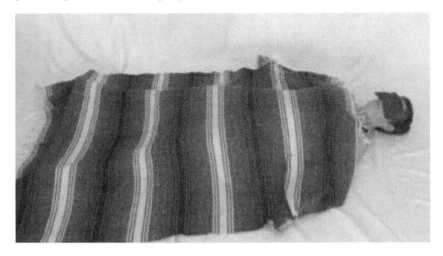

Cover up with a blanket for warmth.

Variations:

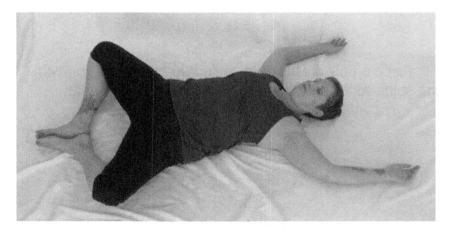

If straight legs are uncomfortable for the low back, try a variation for the legs. Bring the soles of the feet together and allow the knees to fall open for a Butterfly variation.

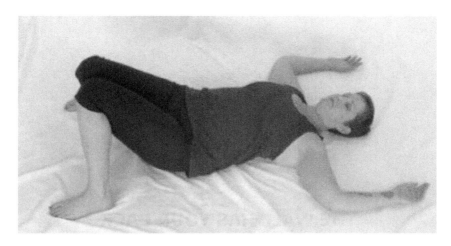

Another variation to support the back is bending the knees and placing the feet on the mat. Separate the feet wider than the hips and allow the knees to rest upon each other.

THE WALL HAS YOUR BACK
(OR YOUR LEGS)

The wall can serve as your ultimate Yin prop for stability. When you take your Yin poses to the wall you may find your body surrenders to the poses on a new level. The wall is strong and sturdy. You need not worry about the wall shifting or changing. Your mind can rest easy knowing that the wall will hold up the body.

Many of the wall poses are done while lying on the back. The mat offers the same strong and sturdy support as the wall. The combination of the wall and mat may allow the body to come to a deeper place of trust. In that trust the body may deepen further in the poses.

Centering on the Wall

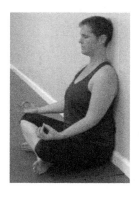

Centering on the wall may bring a fresh perspective to the start of your practice. Place the mat against the wall. Sit in any pose you find comfortable enough to sustain during centering. When I am not at the wall, I normally find my centering position by sitting on blocks in firm pose. When I am centering on the wall, I sit in easy pose with no blocks. Some students sit on a folded blanket with the legs extended in front of the body. The support of the wall may change the way you find comfort in your seat.

Sit close enough to the wall to bring the hips and shoulders to touch the wall. There is a natural curve of the spine that creates a little space between your low back and the wall. Feel the way the shoulders touch the wall. Drawing the shoulders back and down may allow the shoulders to flatten against the wall as you sit. You may want to bring the back of the head to rest against the wall. The hands may come to a comfortable spot on the knees or thighs. Feel free to add a mudra with the hands.

When you have created a space that seems right, start to notice how you feel. You may discover new sensations by centering on the wall. Feel the temperature of the wall on the skin. Notice the way the back of the body moves against the wall with the breath. This may bring greater awareness to the breath. Let this awareness inspire new feelings of being grounded and present. Feel more connected to your body.

Neck Bend

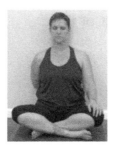 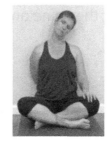

If you are centering on the wall, your body is already in position for a nice stretch in the upper shoulder and neck. Begin this Neck Bend by sitting in a comfortable position with the back against the wall. Bring the right arm behind the back. The arm will slide into that little space between the wall and the low back. Let your body weight lean against the wall. This may create a nice sensation in the shoulder. Stop here if this is enough.

Begin to bring the left ear toward the left shoulder to stretch through the right side of the neck. The sensation may change a bit as the head rolls back toward the wall or gently shifts forward toward the chest. The neck is a very sensitive part of the body so be very mindful when stretching the neck. Be aware of how much sensation you feel and make sure you go to an appropriate place for your body.

Allow the body to feel supported by the mat and the wall. Let the upper body lean back against the wall so you are using very little effort to remain in the pose. If you are bending the neck, allow the head to feel heavy. Check in with how you feel on the side of the neck and the top of the shoulder. Release tension throughout the upper back all the way to the seat. Feel the legs softening.

To release the pose slowly lift the head back through center. You might stay upright for a few breaths before releasing the arm. Allow the arm to rest beside the body or bring the hand on top of the knee or thigh. Notice sensation in the neck, spine, and shoulders. Repeat the pose on the other side for the same amount of time.

Seated Side Bend

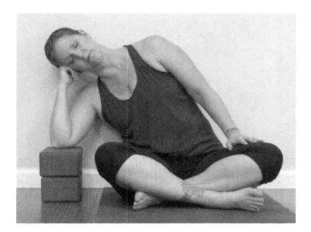

Start from a seated position with the back against the wall. Bring a block or stack of blocks to the right side of the body. Begin to lean the upper body toward the right as the left side of the body begins to open and stretch. Place the right elbow on the block or on the floor. Support the head by making a gentle fist with the right hand. Allow the head to rest against the fist. If this feels like enough sensation, stop here with the left hand resting on the left thigh or waist.

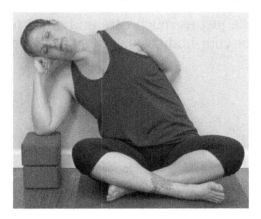

Change the pose a bit by moving the left arm. Try a half bind by bringing the left arm behind the back. The arm will go in the little space between the back and the wall. Let the upper body lean back against the wall.

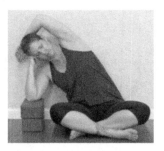

The pose may feel deeper through the side of the body with the left arm overhead. Bring the left arm up and over and allow it to rest on the head. Release the arm if there is too much strain in the neck or shoulders.

As you settle into the pose, begin to notice where you feel sensation in your body. Begin to scan from the hip on the left side of the body. Feel the space between the ribs. If the arm is in a half bind, begin to notice sensation in the shoulder. If the arm is overhead, begin to search for a stretch in the triceps. Let the side of the body soften into the pose.

Be sure to balance the body by taking the pose to the other side. Take just as much care and effort to find the perfect spot for your body to experience the pose on the opposite side.

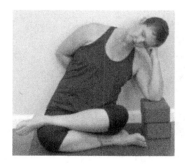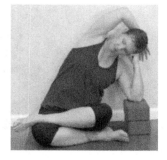

I normally do Seated Side Bend from easy pose where the shins are crossed. If you wanted to add an extra bit of stress to the hips, you could try a different position for the legs. For a deeper sensation you may arrange the legs as you would in Square. If you are opening the right side of the body, bring the left ankle on top of the right knee in Square. When the legs are positioned and you are sitting up tall, begin to work into the Seated Side Bend.

Notice the difference in the pose by simply changing the position of the legs. The hips may feel as if they are stressing a bit more than in easy pose. Change the legs when you are ready to bend on the opposite side.

Bending Branch on the Wall

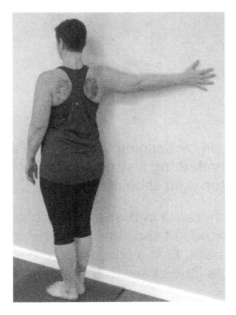

Begin Bending Branch on the Wall by facing the wall. Step close enough to the wall so that you are almost touching it. Bring the right arm out wide with the palm of the hand on the wall. Begin to walk the toes toward the side of the room while the right arm stays in place. The body is gently leaning toward the wall.

If that is not enough sensation on the right shoulder, walk the toes toward the center of the room. The sensation in the shoulder may also change when the arm is adjusted. Try brining the hand a little higher than the shoulder to deepen the shoulder opener. Bring the hand down the wall a few inches to lessen the intensity.

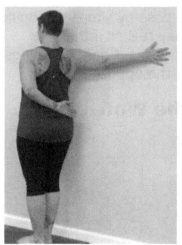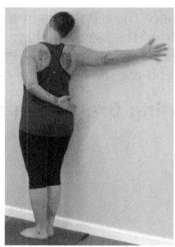

Add a variation by bringing the opposite arm behind the body for a half bind. Bring a stretch to the neck by dropping the right ear to the right shoulder.

Notice the difference in the way the right shoulder feels in comparison to the left shoulder. Feel the sensations in the neck and upper back. Find a space where both shoulders can soften. Lean a little closer to the wall as the body yields to the pose.

Exit the pose by standing away from the wall. Release the arm from the wall. Allow the arm to dangle at the side of the body in stillness for a few breaths.

Repeat on the opposite side for the same amount of time.

Dangle on the Wall

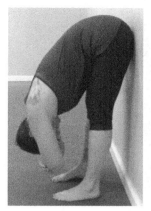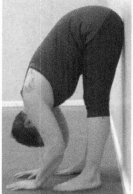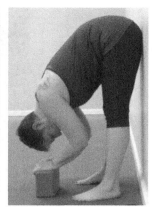

Dangle on the Wall can be done with the buttocks resting on the wall. Begin by standing with the feet hip width apart and the wall a few inches behind you. Begin to walk the hands down the legs into Dangle. Knees start out in a bent position. Begin to straighten the legs to a point of sensation but not pain. Catch opposite elbows to rag doll in the pose or let the hands rest on the floor. Hands can rest on a block for more support.

Do your best to allow the upper body to completely soften. Feel the shoulder blades slide off of the upper back. Allow the head to hang heavy and the neck to feel a bit longer. Let the wall support the body in a way that brings relief to the low back. Feel tension release from behind the legs.

Release the pose by putting a bend in the knees and walking the hands up the legs. Stop at any point if you feel dizzy or light headed. Slowly make your way to a standing position. The body can rest against the wall until you are ready to stand on your own.

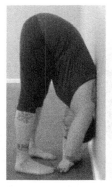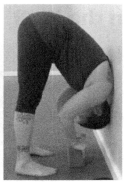

Dangle on the Wall can be done with the upper back resting on the wall. Begin by standing with the wall about a foot in front of you (the distance from the wall will vary from person to person). Make your way into the fold allowing the upper back to rest on the wall. Adjust the feet closer or farther from the wall to find the right space.

Notice if the shoulders are pressing into the wall and creating an uncomfortable bend in the neck. Try to bring the upper back against the wall so the neck is not strained. Adjust the body so that there is comfort in the neck.

This variation may bring more sensation to the back of the legs. Use a block under the hands or bend the knees to soften. Leave the pose if there is pain.

While in the pose bring awareness to the backs of the legs. Allow the legs to feel as if they are lengthening from your heels to the tops of your hamstrings. Feel space in the low back. Notice how the upper back feels against the wall. Lean a little closer to the wall as the body surrenders to the pose.

To leave Dangle on the Wall shift weight into the heels so that the body comes away from the wall. Bend the knees and slowly start to walk the body to an upright position. Bring a hand to the wall to steady the body until you are ready to stand on your own.

Down Dog on the Wall

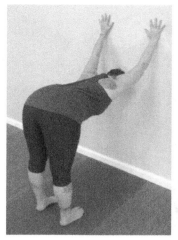 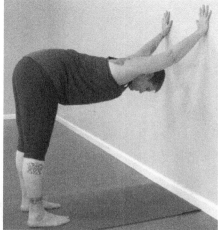

Start Down Dog on the Wall by facing the wall. Stand about two or three feet away from the wall. Adjust the amount of space to suite your body. Bring the hands on to the wall. Make sure the hands are higher than the shoulders. Begin to hinge from the hips and lean forward. Allow the heart to sink toward the floor. The head may drop if there is no strain for the neck.

Begin to feel into the shoulders. Adjust the hands and feet until you can comfortably come into stillness and maintain sensation in the pose. Find that space in you that is feeling the most from the pose. Allow that part of the body to soften on the next exhale. As the most intense place finds ease, begin to explore the rest of the body. Balance the effort and ease of the pose.

To release the pose begin to slowly walk forward and lift the upper body. The hands can stay on the wall as long as you like while the body acclimates to standing. Bring the arms to rest at the sides of the body in stillness for a few breaths.

Prayer Squat on the Wall

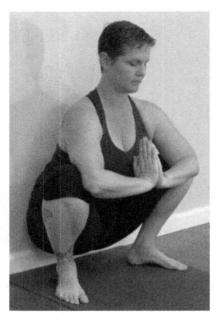

Begin Prayer Squat on the Wall by standing a few inches away from the wall. Begin to bend the knees and slide down the wall. Point the toes in the same direction as the knees. Feel the low back resting against the wall and bring the hands into a prayer position at the heart.

Position the elbows to the inside of the knees. As the palms press toward one another, the elbows may gently press the knees out. This may create a deeper opening for the hips and inner thighs.

Allow the hips to soften into the pose. The wall will support some of the weight of the body as hips sink toward the floor. Begin to notice sensation in the inner thighs. Check in with the knees and ankles. Soften the shoulders and neck as the hips continue to open.

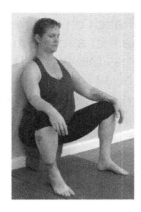

If Prayer Squat on the Wall creates too much pressure for the hips, knees, or ankles, use blocks. Use one or more blocks stacked against the wall. The buttocks will rest on the blocks to take some of the pressure out of the joints.

Twisted Branch on the Wall

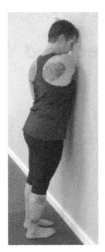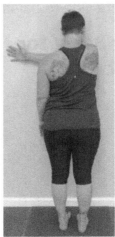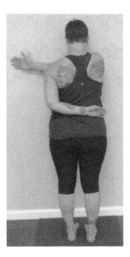

Twisted Branch on the Wall pairs nicely with Bending Branch on the Wall. The poses work the shoulders in opposite directions. One may be done after the other during a sequence.

To enter Twisted Branch on the Wall, begin by facing the wall. Stand with the feet a few inches from the wall. Bring the right arm across the chest. The right palm may touch the wall or face away from the wall. Begin to lean the weight of the body toward the wall. The forehead may lean against the wall if that feels comfortable for the neck. The opposite arm may slide behind the back for a half bind.

Begin to notice how your right shoulder feels. Feel the space behind your shoulder blade. Allow the right upper back to soften in the pose. Let go of tension you may feel in the upper shoulders and neck. Soften all the way down the spine to the low back and buttocks. Allow the body weight to sink into the wall.

Let go of the pose by bringing weight into the heels of the feet. Shift the body away from the wall and allow the arms to rest beside the body. Stand in Mountain Pose as you feel the effects from the pose.

Repeat on the opposite side to balance the body.

Positioning Your Body for Reclined Wall Poses on the Mat

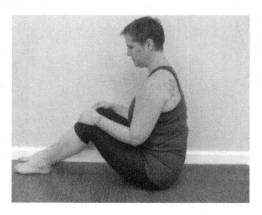

There are many ways to set the body up for reclined wall poses. This is the easiest way I have found to get the body into the right spot. Start by placing the mat next to the wall. Sit on the long edge of the mat with the hip right next to the wall. Lean back toward the mat and at the same time sweep your legs up the wall.

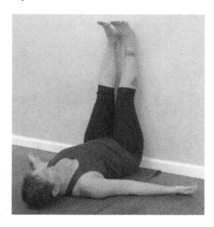

The body is in the middle of the mat. The hips are close to the wall. From this position you will be able to come into the following Yin poses on the wall.

Butterfly on the Wall

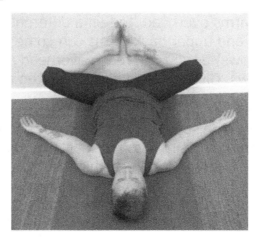

Bring the soles of the feet together. Bend the knees and

allow the heels to come toward the floor. Your body will determine how close the feet should be to the floor. The arms can rest on the mat beside the body. If there is too much sensation in this pose, try scooting the body away from the wall a few inches.

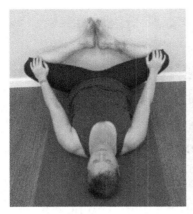 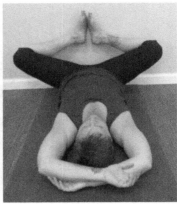

To feel more sensation in the hips and thighs, try pressing the hands against the knees. Press the knees toward the wall. Try to release tension through the shoulders and back when taking this variation. Find balance between the effort you use to press the knees away and the softening the body.

Take the arms overhead to feel a different sensation in the shoulders and upper back. Arms can come to cactus (bend the elbows) or you can reach overhead and hold opposite elbows. Give the body time to soften a bit more through the shoulders in this variation.

Start to feel the support of the mat and the wall. Let the back side of the body sink into the mat. Feel the feet resting against the wall. Soften the inner thighs. Notice the opening in the hips. Search the body for any remaining tension. Let the tension slip away. Notice the inner thighs ease into a more open space as you hold the pose.

Bring the body out of the pose by bringing the knees

together. You may want to take the hands behind the knees and guide them to touch one another. Enjoy the stillness for a few breaths.

Dragonfly on the Wall

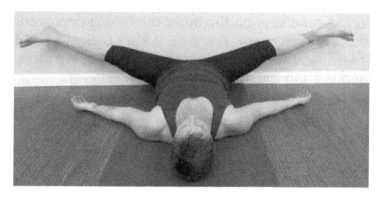

Take a position at the wall to prepare for Dragonfly on the Wall. Straighten the legs and allow the feet to fall in opposite directions. Just allow gravity to find the right amount of space for the legs in this pose. The arms can rest beside the body with the palms facing up.

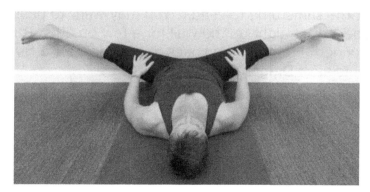

For a deeper sensation in the hips and thighs, bring the hands to rest on the inner thighs. Let the gentle weight from the hands encourage a deeper opening.

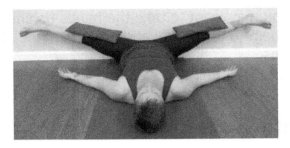

Placing sandbags on the inner thighs will encourage the hips to open even more. It can be a little tricky to find the exact placement for the sandbags without having them fall off. Try adjusting the sandbags to a few different places on the legs to find the right spot.

Let gravity and time do all of the work in this pose. Notice if there is tension in the inner thighs or hips. Feel the sensation in the buttocks and low back. Let the body soften in the understanding that the wall and the mat are supporting the body. Over time notice that the heels come closer to the floor with no physical effort.

After giving way in this pose, the body will need support to leave the posture. Bring the hands to the back of the knees or thighs. Bring one leg at a time to center or both legs at the same time to center. You may want to pause with the legs straight up the wall for a few breaths. It may feel wonderful to bring the knees to the chest for a few moments after Dragonfly on the Wall.

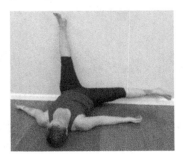

Half Dragonfly on the Wall may bring this pose into a

new place for the body. If the body is tight, this may be a softer variation. If the hips are open, this variation may allow the body to settle more on one side.

Bring both legs up the wall. Allow just the right foot to fall toward the floor. The opposite hip may lift and take some of the sensation from the pose. Try to keep both hips on the floor. Let the arms rest on the floor beside the body.

As the hips release tension, the foot falls closer to the floor. Feel the inner thigh lengthen without struggle. Soften the buttocks and low back. Feel the way the mat supports the body from the crown of the head all the way down to the tailbone. Release the body completely into the pose.

Release the pose by bringing the right foot up to meet the left foot. Pause for a few breaths with both legs straight. Counter the pose here or take the pose on the opposite side.

Frog on the Wall

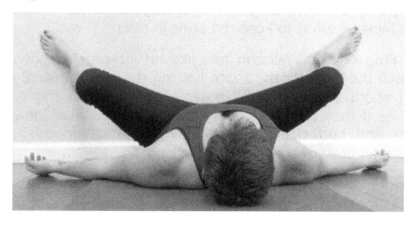

Begin the pose by bending the knees so that the knees are right in line with the ankles. Begin to heel toe the feet apart. The feet will come apart in the shape of a half circle or a rainbow. The feet separate and come closer to the floor as the body deepens into the pose. Slide the body away from the wall to reduce intensity in the pose.

Come into stillness when there is enough sensation in the hips and inner thighs. Allow the arms to rest beside the body.

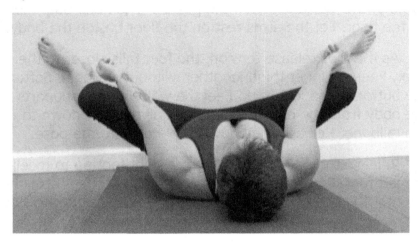

To bring more sensation to the inner thighs and hips, try placing the forearms on the inner thighs or knees. Allow the weight of the arms to gently encourage a deeper opening. Use minimal effort to keep the arms in place.

Frog on the Wall can feel like an intense hip opener. Search the body for the space holding the most tension. Let that space soften into the pose. Allow the inner thighs to feel as if they are lengthening. Bring awareness to the low back and buttocks. Feel the way the mat supports the backside of the body without asking for assistance from muscular strength. Find ease in the stillness.

Come out of the pose by heel toeing the feet back together. Pause for a moment when the feet and knees are touching. After a few breaths extend the legs.

Spinal Twist on the Wall

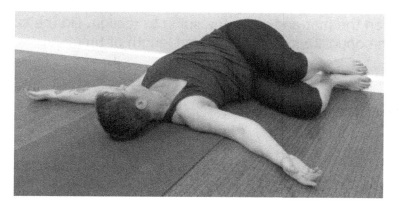

With the legs straight up the wall, bend the knees and walk the feet down the wall until the shins are parallel to the floor. Feel the entire backside on the mat. Feel the way the shoulders and hips lay evenly on the mat. Shift the hips slightly to the left. Begin to walk the feet and knees over to the right. The right knee and the edge of the right foot may touch the floor. Notice how the hips started to align so that the left hip stacks on the right hip. The shoulders stay connected to the floor with the arms outstretched.

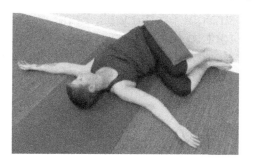

A sandbag may help deepen the twist. Place the sandbag on the upper thigh of the top leg.

Begin to settle into the pose. Soften all along the spine from the neck to the tailbone. Feel the gentle twist in the spine. Search for tension in the shoulders and hips. Allow the body to soften into the pose. Settle into stillness.

Let go of the twist by coming back through center. Walk the feet back to their original location. Bring both hips to rest on the mat and allow the spine to realign. Do the same on the opposite side for the same length of time.

Tree on the Wall

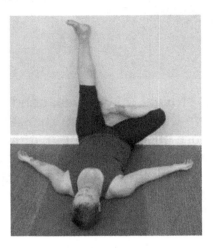

Tree on the Wall can be a very gentle hip opener. Begin with both legs straight up the wall. Bend the right knee. Bring the right foot to the inside of the left leg. Let gravity decide how far down the leg to place the foot. The right knee gently leans toward the wall.

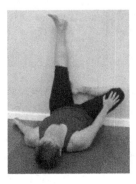

For a little added sensation, press the knee toward the

wall. Take the right hand and press on the knee until the right amount of sensation is felt in the hip.

This pose may not bring a great deal of stress for the body. Focus on letting go of tension throughout the body a bit more. Feel the entire backside of the body from the back of the head all the way to the buttocks resting comfortably on the mat. Feel the firm support from the earth. Notice softening through the hips. Feel lengthening on the back side of the straight leg. Enjoy the support of this pose.

Leave the pose by straightening the bent knee. Take a few breaths with both legs straight up the wall. Repeat on the other side when the body is ready.

Square on the Wall

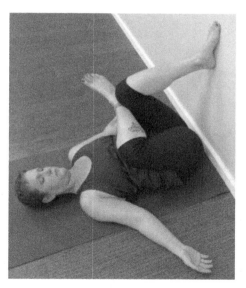

Square on the Wall is a personal favorite of mine. This is a wonderful hip opener. From Legs Up the Wall, bend the knees until the ankles are in line with the knees. Press through the feet to lift the hips. Bring the right ankle to rest on the left knee and very slowly begin to lower the hips back down to the mat. If the hips do not comfortably come to the mat, scoot the body away from the wall a few inches.

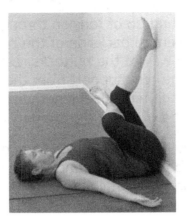

If there is too much pressure on the hips, begin to straighten the left leg. The body will feel greater ease in the pose the more the leg is straightened.

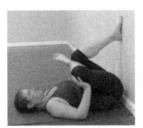

To find a bit more intensity in the pose, place the right hand on the right knee. Begin to slowly press the knee toward the wall. Try to isolate the muscular engagement to the arm while the rest of the body releases into the pose.

Begin to identify the feelings in the right hip. Let the hip soften. Spread your awareness throughout the body. Soften the buttocks and low back. Feel the shoulders settle against the mat. Breathe into the stillness of the pose.

Leave the pose the same way you entered. Press the left foot against the wall enough to lift the hips. Release the right foot to the wall and slowly lower the hips to the mat. Rest for a few moments with the back flat on the mat and the feet on the wall. Straighten the legs when the body is ready.

Repeat on the other side to balance the body.

Legs Up the Wall

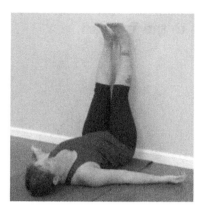

Legs Up the Wall is such a restful pose it can be the Savasana pose for a Yin on the Wall class. The legs are resting on the wall while the arms are stretched out wide. Scoot the hips away from the wall to find a bit more effortlessness.

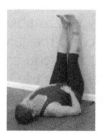 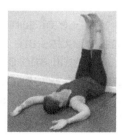 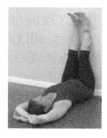

The hands can rest on the belly to connect to the breath and soften the shoulders. For a different sensation in the shoulders, bring the arms overhead. You can try cactus arms with the elbows bent or reach overhead bringing the hands to the elbows.

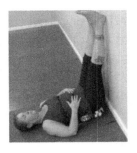

Try a blanket under the low back. This will lift the hips and bring softness to the low back.

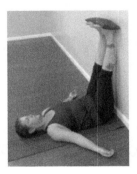

Place a weight on the feet for a variation of this pose. A sandbag or two on top of the feet will help the body feel grounded in this position. The sandbags can provide a space for the body to use less effort and find more comfort.

When your body has found the right arrangement, become still. Come into a place of serenity where absolutely nothing moves. All of the muscles are soft and the joints are feeling spacious. Become so still and quiet that you can feel and hear your heart beating in your chest. Allow the body to be completely free from stress and tension. Feel entirely present in both mind and body.

Leave the pose when you are ready by bending the knees and rolling to the side. You may place your arm under your head and stay here for a few breaths. Use the hands to gently press yourself up into your seat. Stay seated until the body is ready to move.

COUNTERING THE POSES

I believe there is some debate in the Yin yoga world about countering each Yin pose with movement. I am in the camp in favor of countering poses. I have watched people practice Yin for years and it seems they respond to movement after each pose. It's as if the body needs some movement to reset the body after stillness. It generally takes less than a minute to create space for the next pose.

Immediately after each pose there is stillness. The body is still so that you can absorb the effects of the pose. Energy is moving and shifting as a result of the posture. Remain still for a few breaths or as long as you are "feeling" the pose. Remember that one of the benefits of Yin yoga is to balance the chi or energy that is moving through the meridian lines of the body. Let your body have a chance to get the chi moving.

When the body is ready to move, let your body be your guide. Yin yoga is an intimate and deeply personal practice. You are training yourself to listen to the body during this practice. You listen to the body during the pose. You listen to your body after the pose as you are in stillness. And you listen to the body after stillness for cues on how to move.

There is a natural instinct to start to move. Listen to that natural feeling. If you are not sure what movements to take, let me offer a few suggestions.

After a pose that allows the spine to round forward such as Caterpillar, the body may want to counter with a pose that moves the spine into length or into a back bend. Take a seated back bend by bringing the hands onto the mat behind you. Press down through the palms and the sits bones as the chest lifts toward the sky. Squeeze the shoulder blades together to lift the heart a little higher.

Twists are also a nice way to counter forward folds. You could take an informal seated twist by stacking the spine and twisting to each side. If the body needs the twist to feel a little deeper come into a seated twist (Ardha Matsyendrasana) by bringing the right foot to the outside of the left knee. The left arm can wrap around the knee or the left elbow can come to the outside of the right knee. The right hand will rest on the ground or come to the low back. Do the same twisting to the opposite side.

If you would like a pose which uses a little more strength to counter a forward fold, try Reverse Table Top or Reverse Plank. Reverse Table Top begins from a seated position. Bend the knees so the feet are flat on the mat. Place the hands on the mat behind you. Press down through the feet and hands to lift the hips in line with the knees and shoulders.

Reverse Plank is very similar to Reverse Table Top. From a seated position the legs are extended in front of the body. Hands are on the mat behind the body. Press down through the heels and palms to lift the hips. This pose is sometimes called Upward Plank as it looks just like plank facing up.

Hips are often the focus of Yin poses. Be still for a

moment after the hip opener. When you are ready to move, listen to your body to guide you into countering the pose.

After a hip opener it may feel good to windshield wiper the knees. Sit on the mat with the knees bent. The feet are flat on the mat and can be spaced a little farther apart than the hips. Hands are on the mat behind the body. Slowly sway the knees form side to side.

Maybe the body is craving a pose that requires more strength after a hip opener. Downward Facing Dog often feels pretty good after a pose like Swan and Sleeping Swan. Bring movement to this Downward Facing Dog by pedaling out the legs (walk your dog) or swaying the hips from side to side (wag your tail). Try a Three Legged Dog from Down Dog. Lift one leg to the sky then stack the hips and bend the knee.

Child's Pose with the knees close together can feel especially nice after a pose like Dragonfly or Frog. The arms can be outstretched with fingers reaching forward or the arms may rest alongside the body. Try swaying the hips slightly from side to side to relieve any pressure in the low back or hips.

If the knees were bent in the hip opener like in Square Pose or Butterfly it may feel good to the body to stretch out the legs. Start from a seated position and stretch the heels toward the front of the mat. You might like to reach toward the toes or hold on to the ankles to give the back of the legs a little extra stretch.

These counters are just suggestions. You may find that your body requires a different way to move after a Yin pose. Listening to and responding to your body is the best counter pose.

YIN YOGA SEQUENCES

Now that you know many of the Yin Yoga poses, you may wonder how to put the poses together to create a class. I often have a theme that guides me through which poses to choose to sequence a class. The theme may center around a feeling, a quote, a chakra, a meridian pair, a season, or whatever strikes my fancy for that day.

I would like to share some of my thoughts on how I put together specific sequences. Try one of these classes or use the sequences as inspiration to build your own.

Spleen/Stomach Meridian Practice

One morning I was feeling very tired. My body was lacking energy and motivation. I wanted to come up with some poses that might help me feel better. I began thinking about which meridian is are associated with helping to uplift energy levels. When the spleen meridian is out of balance, the body may feel fatigued.

The Yang organ that pairs with the spleen is stomach. In TCM the spleen is said to contain the body's thoughts and intentions. When the energy or chi in the spleen and stomach are in balance a person may physically improve digestion. Improved digestion may allow the body to properly absorb the nutrients from the food that you eat. These nutrients help to fuel the body and boost energy.

I decided to put together a few poses that would help to balance spleen and stomach meridians energy with the hope of increasing energy and feeling better.

Start the sequence with Centering then bring the body into the following poses.

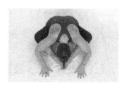

Butterfly

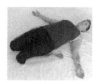

Saddle

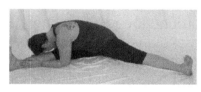

Dragonfly-lean over the leg

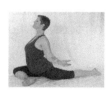

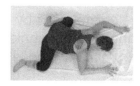

Swan

Frog

Spinal Twist

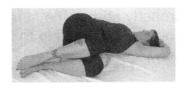

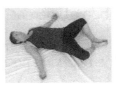

Recline Butterfly or Legs up the Wall

Savasana

Liver/Gallbladder Meridian and Heart Chakra Practice

I watched a movie and I was struck by what one of the characters said at the end of the movie. The line was something like, "with a little love and courage, we can change the world." This inspired me to create a class around love and kindness. The liver and gallbladder meridians are associated with balancing emotions and compassion. The heart chakra is the source of love, caring, and nurturing. I focused on the liver and gallbladder meridian lines and the heart chakra for this class. During centering, I encouraged students to focus on Love and Kindness meditation.

To practice Love and Kindness meditation you will start with centering. Find a comfortable seat and begin to quiet the mind by closing the eyes and focusing on the inhales and exhales. As the mind and body begin to settle you can say these four lines to yourself:

- May I be safe.
- May I be happy.
- May I be healthy.
- May I walk on the earth in peace.

This meditation practice always begins with sending love and kindness to yourself first. You must have a full heart before sending love and kindness to others. Self care is important if you want to share your energy with others.

As your heart begins to feel full, you may change the object of your love and kindness. You might put another person's name in place of "I." This person may be someone that you are close to. It may be someone you want to receive your loving and kind energy to brighten their day.

Sometimes the object of this meditation is a person who is in need. This person may be feeling a little down or be physically ill. You can send your positive vibes their way during this practice.

It may seem strange, but you can also focus on a person or group that you do not like during this meditation. If you are trying to let go of anger or negative feelings, Love and Kindness meditation can be a valuable tool. Place the person's name in the meditation and watch as your heart begins to soften in their direction. This variation of the meditation reminds me of a quote from Martin Luther King Jr. "Darkness cannot drive out darkness; only light can do that. Hate cannot drive out hate; only love can do that."

You might end your love and kindness meditation by sending out your loving energy to all beings. Wishing that all those on the planet feel a little better because you are sending them your good intentions.

After centering, you may sit in stillness for a moment longer before moving on to the poses. Try a few of these poses while keeping the uplifting energy from your love and kindness practice close to your heart.

Start the sequence with Love and Kindness Meditation then bring the body into the following poses.

Butterfly

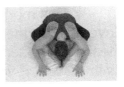

Recline Butterfly

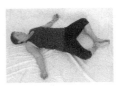

Seated Head to Knee

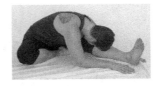

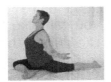 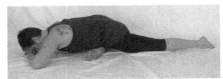

Swan

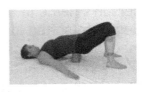

Supported Bridge

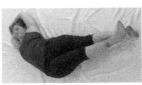

Bananasana

Savasana

Chakra Practice

From time to time I do a meditation practice that focuses on aligning the chakras. During this meditation, I focus on each chakra starting with the root chakra. I focus on the color of the chakra and how I can feel when the chakras are balanced and the chi is flowing freely. This meditation always leaves me feeling energized and strong.

I decided to create a Yin practice that would focus on a single chakra in each pose. During the class I think about each chakra that is targeted in the pose. I think about the light and energy in each chakra glowing brighter and brighter. I try to feel the location of the chakra in my body. My goal is to let go of anything that might be blocking the energy of the chakras.

As you center, you may focus on the breath moving up and down your spine. The chakras are aligned along the spine. Imaging that your breath begins at the base of your spine. Visualize a ball of light at the base of the spine. As you breathe, the ball moves up the spine. At the top of the breath, the ball of light is at the crown of the head. The ball of light moves back toward the base of the spine on the exhale. Repeat until the mind and body have settled.

Try this sequence to balance your chakras.

Caterpillar - Focus on the root chakra also called the Muladhara chakra. This chakra is red. It is located at the base of the spine in the first three vertebrae. The root chakra is the chakra of stability, security, and survival issues. When in balance you feel safe and fearless.

Butterfly - Focus on the sacral chakra also known as the Svadhisthana chakra. This chakra is orange and located above the pubic bone and below the belly button. The sacral chakra is associated with creativity, pleasure, and sexuality. When in balance you may feel more creative and able to enjoy the pleasures life has to offer.

Spinal Twist - The third chakra is the solar plexus chakra or the Manipura chakra. This chakra is yellow and is located from the belly button to the breastbone. It is known as the chakra of power, self worth, and self-confidence. When flowing freely you may feel complete satisfaction and contentment.

Melting Heart - Focus on the fourth chakra which is the heart chakra. The heart chakra is green and also called the Anahata chakra. This chakra is located in the center of the breastbone. It is the source of love, caring, nurturing, and connection. When the heart chakra is balanced you feel love for yourself and others even in tough times.

Supported Fish - The fifth chakra is the throat chakra. The throat chakra is also called the Vishuddha chakra. It is light blue. The chakra is located in the throat including the neck, thyroid, jaw, mouth, and tongue. It is the chakra of diplomacy. The throat chakra is the source of self expression and the ability to speak our highest truth. When this chakra is flowing freely you will speak clearly with truth.

Wide Knee Child's Pose - with the third eye resting on a block, the mat, or the back of the hands - The sixth chakra is the third eye chakra or the Anja chakra. It is located on the forehead between the eyebrows. It is indigo in color. This is the center of intuition, imagination, and wisdom. When in balance you can see clearly into your heart and soul.

Square - Focus on the seventh chakra know as the crown chakra or the Sahaswara chakra. This chakra is violet and located at the crown of the head. This is the source of enlightenment and bliss. When flowing freely there is a spiritual connection to our higher selves, to others, and to the Devine.

Savasana

Fall Practice

There are times when the season inspires what I want to practice. Fall is associated with the lung and large intestine meridians. When the lung meridian is out of balance one my feel sad. When this meridian is in balance you may feel your thinking is clear. Balanced lung and large intestine meridians may lead to a positive self image, a happy outlook, and the ability to loosen up and let go. The function of the lungs is to breathe life giving air into the body. The lung meridian brings new chi or energy to the body. The function of the large intestine is to let go of waste. The large intestines meridian allows you to energetically let go of what is no longer serving you. Just as the trees release the leaves in the fall, a person can view the season of fall as a time to let go.

Start the sequence with Centering then bring the body into the following poses.

Dangle

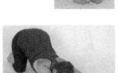

Melting Heart - Quarter Dog variation

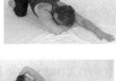

Dragonfly with lateral stretch

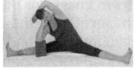

Sphinx with an additional minute in Seal

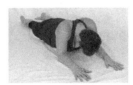

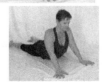

Butterfly

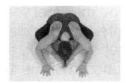

Square with optional Eagle Arms

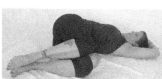

Spinal Twist

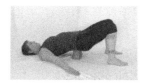

Supported Bridge

Savasana

Santosha Practice

I'm often struck by a feeling like joy or a concept like santosha. Santosha is a Sanskrit word that means contentment or complete satisfaction. I decided to theme a class around santosha and chose to use poses that bring peace and contentment both to my mind and body. If the following sequence does not bring feelings of contentment and satisfaction to your mind and body, you could create your own sequence by imagining what feels amazing to your body.

Start the sequence with Centering then bring the body into the following poses.

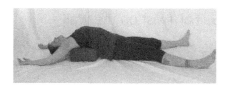

Supported Fish

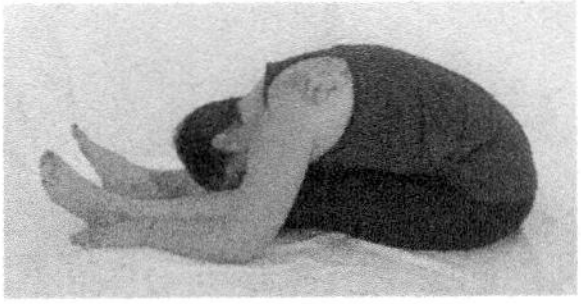

Caterpillar

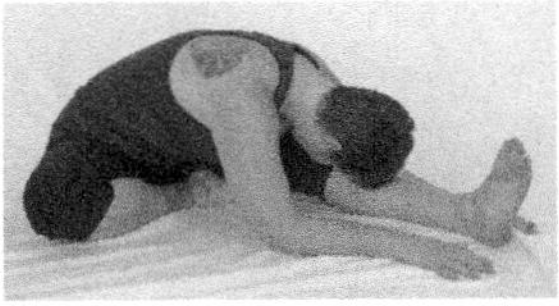

Seated Head to Knee

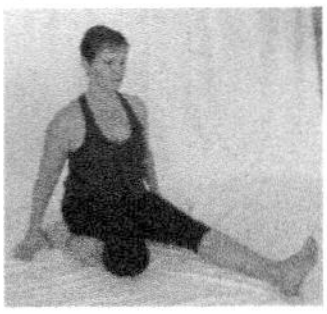

Half Saddle

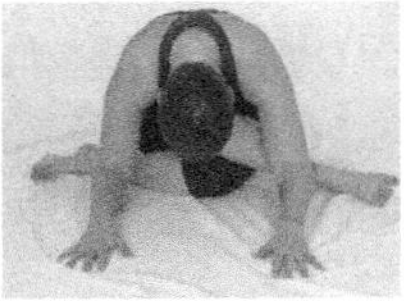

Shoelace

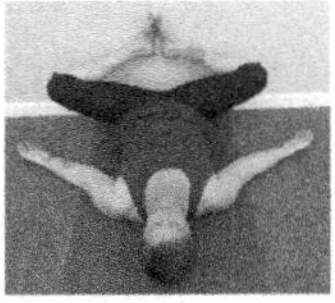

Butterfly on the Wall

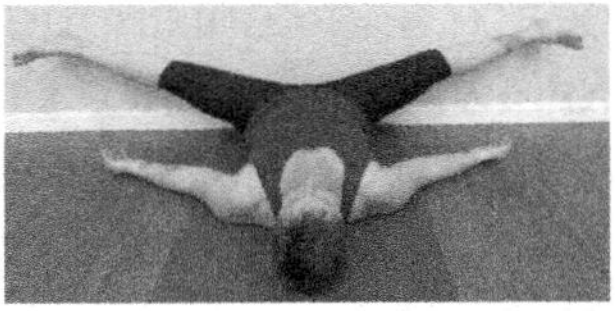

Dragonfly on the Wall

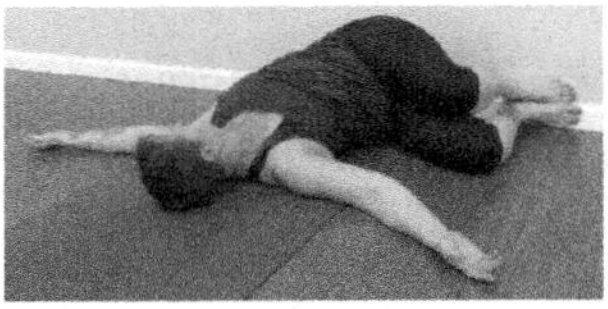

Spinal Twist on the Wall

Legs Up the Wall can serve as Savasana

Hip Opening Practice

I love it when students make requests. I am happy to create a class that will help someone feel better. Often, the requests center around a part of their body that feels tight. Most often I hear requests to open the hips. For those students who are tight in the hips, it's important to think about using props. Props may allow a student to get more out of the poses.

Start the sequence with Centering then bring the body into the following poses.

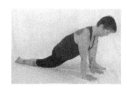

Dragon-try one of the variations

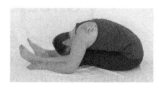

Caterpillar

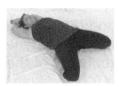

Reverse Wide Knee Child's Pose

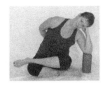

Square with lateral stretch

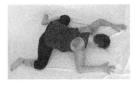

Frog

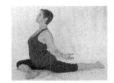 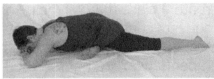

Swan

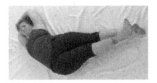

Bananasana

Savasana

Shoulder Opening Practice

Sometimes, students request poses to open the upper back. Imagine how many hours each day you spend hunching forward over a keyboard. If you have a long commute, your hands are attached to the steering wheel and the shoulders may round forward for a good part of the day. Cell phones have brought a new level of sustained rounding of the upper back and bowing the head forward in our community. Put all of these activities together and we have a population that is crying out for upper back and neck relief.

Start the sequence with Centering then bring the body into

the following poses.

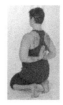

Toe Squat with a grip from behind

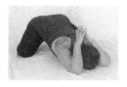

Wide Knee Child's Pose with the thumbs to the back of the neck

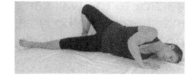

Bending Branch

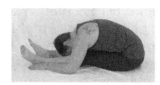

Caterpillar

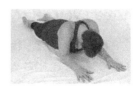

Sphinx

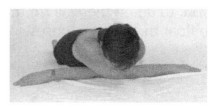

Twisted Branches

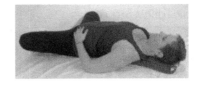

Recline Butterfly with a blanket along the spine

Savasana

Yin on the Wall Practice

I wanted to create a class that centered on the concept of trust. When our bodies trust us and we trust our bodies, we can enter a new level of stillness in Yin poses. Taking the practice to the wall can supply a tangible place that is strong and sturdy. The body can physically trust that the mat and the wall will shore up the body.

I was looking for inspirational words about trust when I came across Alan Watts. Alan Watts was a philosopher who explained Eastern philosophies to a Western audience. I was struck by a quote by him. Watts said, "To have faith is to trust yourself to the water. When you swim you don't grab hold of the water, because if you do you will sink and drown. Instead you relax, and float."

It is easy to have faith in what you see with the eyes. You can see the wall. You can see the mat. Have faith that your body is completely supported. The muscles have no work to do on the wall. In that faith and trust allow the body to float through the poses.

Start by Centering on the Wall

Seated Side Bend on the Wall

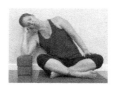

Down Dog on the Wall

Bending Branch on the Wall

Twisting Branch on the Wall

Dangle on the Wall

Prayer Squat on the Wall with blocks

Butterfly on the Wall

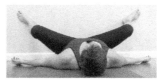

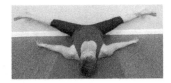

Dragonfly on the Wall

Frog on the Wall

Square on the Wall

Legs up the Wall-this may be used as Savasana

Many thanks to all who contributed to the making of this book.I could not have done this without the talented photography of my husband, Michael Blei.

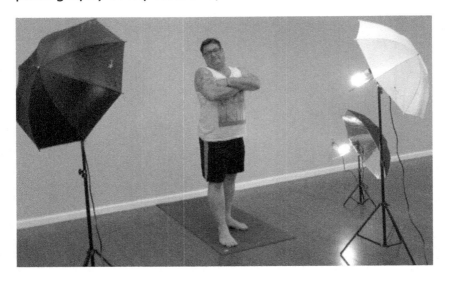

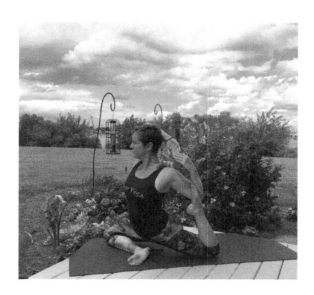

About the Author

Sue Blei has been teaching in some fashion for most of her life. She transitioned from teaching first grade students to teaching yoga to opening her own yoga studio and teaching others how to teach yoga. Serving others by leading them to their own truth has been a lifelong mission for Sue. And then she found Yin.

Made in the USA
Middletown, DE
05 August 2019